Practitioner Research in Health Care

Edited by

Jan Reed

and

Sue Procter

*Senior Lecturers
at the Institute of Health Sciences
University of Northumbria, Newcastle, UK*

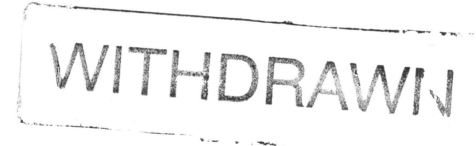
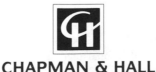

CHAPMAN & HALL

London · Glasgow · Weinheim · New York · Tokyo · Melbourne · Madras

Published by Chapman & Hall, 2–6 Boundary Row, London SE1 8HN, UK

Chapman & Hall, 2–6 Boundary Row, London, SE1 8HN, UK

Blackie Academic & Professional, Wester Cleddens Road, Bishopbriggs, Glasgow G64 2NZ, UK

Chapman & Hall GmbH, Pappelallee 3, 69469 Weinheim, Germany

Chapman & Hall Inc., One Penn Plaza, 41st Floor, New York NY 10119, USA

Chapman & Hall Japan, Thomson Publishing Japan, Hirakawacho Nemoto Building 6F, 1–7–11 Hirakawa-cho, Chiyoda-ku, Tokyo 102, Japan

Chapman & Hall Australia, Thomas Nelson Australia, 102 Dodds Street, South Melbourne, Victoria 3205, Australia

Chapman & Hall India, R. Seshadri, 32 Second Main Road, CIT East, Madras 600 035, India

Distributed in the USA and Canada by Singular Publishing Group Inc., 4284 41st Street, San Diego, California 92105

First edition 1995

© 1995 Chapman & Hall

Typeset in 10/12pt Palatino by Florencetype Ltd, Stoodleigh, Devon
Printed in Great Britain by Page Bros, Norwich

ISBN 0 412 49810 3   1 56593 189 0 (USA)

The publisher makes no representation, express or implied, with regard to the accuracy of the information contained in this book and cannot accept any legal responsibility or liability for any errors or omissions that may be made.

A catalogue record for this book is available from the British Library

∞ Printed on acid-free text paper, manufactured in accordance with ANSI/NISO Z39 48–1992 and ANSI/NISO Z39.48–1984 (Permanence of Paper)

Contents

Contributors

Colin Biott Reader in Education, University of Northumbria at Newcastle (UNN). He has held a number of consultancy and advisory positions with education services both nationally and internationally, with some of his consultancy work being carried out in Iceland.

Jean Davies RN RM Research Midwife, Northern Regional Maternity Survey Office currently analysing data from the Northern Regional 1993 Home Birth Survey. Worked for 10 years as Community Midwife on a Newcastle inner city council estate and was responsible for initiating the Newcastle Community Midwifery Care Project.

Dr Bob Heyman Reader in Health Sciences, University of Northumbria at Newcastle. He has led the Postgraduate Diploma and MSc courses in Health and Social Research (now Health Sciences) for health care professionals until his appointment as Reader.

Sarah Huckle At the time of study, which she completed for her PhD, Sarah was working as a Research Assistant at the Institute for Health Sciences at the University of Northumbria at Newcastle. She is now a senior Research Assistant at the same institution.

Ruth McKeown Ruth is currently employed as a Health Promotion Locality manager for a City Challenge Health Promotion Service. At present she is working on a study looking at the experiences of people waiting six months or more for health treatment.

Dr Liz Meerabeau RGN RHV RNT RHVT MBA. Liz Meerabeau has spent 12 years in various posts in nursing and health visitor education in the London area, including three years as Educational Research Officer at St George's School of Nursing, London. At the time of writing this chapter she was Head of the School of Advanced Nursing at NESCOT, Surrey.

Val Pirie RGN RMN. Valerie is a nurse therapist at the Marion Family Centre in Darlington. She works in a multi-disciplinary setting with children and young people experiencing emotional and/or behavioural problems.

Sue Procter RGN. Principal Lecturer in Nursing at the University of Northumbria. Responsible, with Jan Reed, for setting up the practice development route on the MSc Health Sciences course run at the University of Northumbria. Recently she has started working with the Nursing Development Unit at Wansbeck Hospital. Sue is also collaborating with Colin Biott in a multi-centre European research project co-ordinated by CARE at the University of East Anglia.

Jan Reed RGN. Senior Lecturer in Nursing (Research) at the Institute of Health Sciences at UNN, she is currently on secondment to the Centre of Health services research at Newcastle University where she is a Department of Health Post-doctoral Nursing Research Fellow.

Debbie Skeil MRCP. Now a Consultant in Rehabilitation, Ryhope Hospital Sunderland, at the time of the research, she was a Senior Registrar in rehabilitation, Hunters Moor Regional Rehabilitation Centre, Newcastle upon Tyne.

Chris Stevenson RMN. Chris has worked in the field of mental health services, and is currently a Senior Lecturer in Health Studies at the University of Sunderland. She is currently completing her PhD, which studied family therapy processes.

Preface

Health care practitioners have been exhorted by various bodies and authorities over the years to develop 'research-based practice'. The arguments behind these exhortations have generally been that research provides a more sure and certain knowledge, superior to the tacit or traditional knowledge that practitioners build up or inherit in the course of practice. There are, of course, many objections that could be and have been raised against this type of thinking, with its touching faith in the certainties of science and corresponding dismissal of experiential learning, and indeed some of these objections are discussed in this book. We have tried, however, to give more space to another of the problems inherent in the 'research knowledge is best' position, and that is the assumption that practitioners can choose between science and experience; in other words that they can adopt a scientific stance which excludes and forgets any understanding that they have developed during practice.

As practitioner researchers ourselves, we have found this impossible to do. Many of the research decisions that we have made, including our choice of research question, were based on prior experience of practice. This undoubtedly had many advantages – we knew how organizations worked and could negotiate them effectively; we knew how practice happened, and could identify sources of data and anomalies in our analysis. The problem that we had, however, was in writing up this process of using 'insider knowledge' in a way that would make it 'academically respectable' (particularly an issue when the research would be submitted for an academic award).

Related to our guilt about using non-scientific knowledge in rational research decisions was also the feeling that we were vulnerable to accusations of 'subjectivity'. This subjectivity, according to the texts that we read, was something that happened to people who were 'too close' to the field and did not maintain distance. It could lead to terrible things: a 'lack of analytic clarity', 'atheoretical analysis' or, most dreaded of all, 'bias'. To protect ourselves from bias, we endlessly devised research strategies that would minimize the impact of our professional knowledge, and tried to see the world of practice through a stranger's eyes.

Not surprisingly, abandoning our professional knowledge proved extremely difficult and, in addition, we began to wonder if it was really necessary. This concern was confirmed when we began to become involved in supervising other practitioner researchers, and revisited the dilemmas that we had gone through in our own first attempts at research. Despite our reassurances that practitioner knowledge was a valid basis for research (after all, the aim of the research was to contribute to practitioner knowledge) our students were reluctant to 'come clean' in writing about practitioner knowledge, despite the very articulate cases they made for it in verbal discussions. What they wanted, they said, was a reference that they could use to support their decisions – in other words, they did not feel confident enough to write about these issues without referring to the writing of a respected methodologist, someone who would validate their practitioner knowledge.

There was, however, very little to be found in the literature which discussed the ambivalent role of the practitioner researcher, and while this search for references can be regarded as one of the problems inherent in traditional academic assessment criteria, it also highlights a serious gap in methodological literature. Perhaps because other non-professional disciplines (e.g. sociology, psychology, social policy, physiology etc.) have a long research tradition, methodological texts for health care disciplines have tended to borrow from the work done in these other fields, and have not paid much attention to the particular circumstances and goals of practitioner research. As practitioners become more and more involved in research, however, the need for such a discussion becomes more and more pressing.

This book is an attempt to stimulate this debate. It is not a manual for practitioner research, and it contains few instructions or procedures to follow. What we hope it will do is to generate a careful and critical debate about the nature of practitioner research and its relationship to other forms of knowledge. It is not an uncritical defence of practitioner research – we recognize that, like all research, it has limitations and, moreover, that other types of research make different and equally valuable contributions to the knowledge that informs practice. What we do argue, however, is that when practitioners become involved in research, then that research will necessarily involve and use practice-derived knowledge and its aim will primarily be to contribute to practice knowledge. This is not a question of preference or choice: it is the case because it is impossible to forget years of training and practice as soon as one adopts a research role. Given that practitioner researchers have practice experience and research experience, discussing the latter at the expense of the former seems to be a wasteful strategy for developing practice. We cannot afford a situation where practitioners have to deny their practice knowledge in order to contribute to it.

We hope, therefore, that this book will play a part in the development of practitioner research as a distinct form of enquiry, undertaken in particular circumstances by people with particular experiences and goals. Such a development is, however, a long-term project which will involve much work. From our discussions and explorations we have identified a number of areas which require further thought, in particular the nature of practice-based knowledge, the criteria by which practitioner research might be evaluated, the place of values in practitioner research, and the relationship between practice methodology and research methodology – others can probably think of more. Practitioner research, then, is far from cut and dried, and perhaps it never will be. The attempt to examine it more closely, is, we believe, still a worthwhile endeavour. Whether we like it or not, as practitioners, practitioner research is what we do – the choice is whether we do it with some insight or none.

Jan Reed and Sue Proctor
Newcastle upon Tyne
January 1994

PART ONE

Basic Issues in Practitioner Research

CHAPTER 1

Practitioner research in context

Jan Reed and Sue Procter

INTRODUCTION

The problems of practitioner researchers, that is, practitioners who are involved in doing research into areas of their practice, are on first examination no different from those of any other researchers. The issues of methodology, research tools and data collection are, it would appear, universal, whatever the background of the researcher. When planning a research project, therefore, the practitioner researcher will invariably consult methodological texts for information and advice. At some levels this information is adequate – techniques such as statistical analysis, for example, seem to be easily applied to all types of research that require them. In other ways, however, most methodological texts will not be helpful to practitioner researchers, or may even serve to perplex them even more.

This unhelpfulness is apparent when the texts begin to discuss issues such as developing research questions, theory testing and generation or data analysis. There appears to be something that does not quite fit the experience of the practitioner researcher: indeed these texts seem unaware of the existence of this experience. Reading such texts, it might be thought that they were written for researchers who are strangers to, or at least have only a nodding acquaintance with, the world that they are researching. The texts may have examples of research studies which, to the practitioner, seem naive or simplistic because they reveal little acknowledgement of the complexities of the issue being studied. They may discuss issues such as 'gaining familiarity with' or 'entry into' the field, which may seem to the practitioner researcher to be unnecessary. These discussions take place in these texts because they are written for people unfamiliar with the research field – in other words people who are not practitioners but are academic researchers – and therefore reflect the aims, objectives and concerns of academia. This is perfectly appropriate – a sociologist, for example, when all is said and done, is seeking primarily to contribute towards the development of sociology, and whereas there may be 'spin-offs' in the sense that the research may inform practice, informing sociology is the priority.

However, this puts the practitioner researcher in a difficult position. If unfamiliarity (sometimes interpreted as 'objectivity' in some texts) is not only assumed, but also appears to be valued, then what do practitioner researchers do? They cannot possibly achieve this degree of distance from their research unless they can find some way of forgetting their past experiences (and perhaps also ignoring their future), and this would appear to be an impossible feat. Can they ever produce 'good' research then, if their data and analysis are so contaminated by their 'subjective' impressions and opinions?

One strategy that many practitioner researchers appear to attempt, in order to make their research 'scientifically respectable', is to ignore, or fail to reveal, their experience. Research decisions that they actually make on the basis of their prior knowledge of situations and issues are rigorously disguised as scientific decisions, and justified by reference to the methodological literature. It is almost as if experientially gained knowledge and understanding is something which is an embarrassment, rather than a resource for research.

PURE AND APPLIED RESEARCH

This seems to be a tragic waste of knowledge, yet it is difficult to see how practitioner researchers can do otherwise, given that the knowledge they have gained from practice is not regarded as 'scientific' knowledge, and 'science' is the business that practitioner researchers are interested in. Their knowledge might be valued as the topic of someone else's study, but as a resource for their own it is not. This difference in the status of different types of knowledge is also reflected in the way that different types of research have been traditionally regarded, for example the difference in status between pure (high status) and applied (low status) research.

Health care research has been called by some 'applied research', in other words that it is not conducted to develop methodology and theory but to develop practice. It draws upon 'pure' theory and methodology, and in doing so it may well adapt them but has little part in developing them. The theories that health care research draws upon ranges from the 'hard' sciences of biology, physiology, pharmacology and the like, to the 'soft' sciences of sociology, psychology and anthropology. This range of disciplines also represents a range of epistemological positions, in other words, ideas about what is considered valid knowledge and what is considered the correct way to acquire it. These epistemological positions are often debated within the disciplines, but this debate is conducted in order to develop the discipline, and is predicated upon the assumption that only members of the discipline will make a contribution to it and that it will only be relevant to those members. For those outside these disciplines, i.e. health care practitioners, the debate does indeed have little relevance, for it does not encompass their particular situations and research contexts. The position of being a practitioner and a researcher at the same time is not one which has been well served by academic debates.

Practitioner researchers are people who are part of the world that they are researching in a way that an academic researcher cannot be. Academic researchers may become part of a culture for the period of the research, but practitioner researchers are part of the culture both before and afterwards. They have a history and a future in that culture: indeed, this is their culture. Their commitment to developing knowledge and understanding will necessarily be motivated by their position in this culture. This position clearly makes their perspective very different from that of the traditional researcher, and yet they will find little recognition of their problems, or even their existence, in most writing on research methodology.

DEPERSONALIZED RESEARCH

The importance of the researcher in research is an issue that has, of course, been exhaustively debated in methodological texts. The positions adopted *vis à vis* the 'human element' of research have ranged from the negative to the positive. The negative view of the researcher is one which is traditionally associated with the classic method of the 'hard' sciences, for example physics and chemistry. Here the attempt is made to negate the researcher and depersonalize the research. Strict protocol is followed in order to ensure that the research can be replicated by others, and so that it does not matter which individual carries out the data collection or analysis. If the human element is acknowledged, it is regarded as a possible source of 'contamination' in the research, which must be controlled at all costs.

This traditional view of science is, of course, an idealistic one. It may not even be a particularly productive one: many accounts of scientific breakthroughs – for example the discovery of the structure of DNA by Watson and Crick – make it clear that the researchers brought to their work unique knowledge, insight and abilities which did not accord with accepted scientific method, yet made great contributions to understanding. By denying the individuality of the researcher, and by seeking to homogenize research practice, science may be in danger of limiting development.

Another ideal of depersonalized research is that it should stand apart from social and political issues – it should remain 'pure'. Not only should the researcher have no personality or idiosyncratic insights, they should also have no culture or political beliefs. Again, of course, this is nonsense. In a world where research needs funding, this funding is necessarily controlled by bodies which have views about what is or is not acceptable. These views therefore control to a great extent what questions are asked in research and how these should be investigated. Examples of this control are numerous throughout the history of science, from the problems that astronomers had in pursing their studies due to the influence of the church in pre-Renaissance times, to the current debates about funding research into renewable sources of energy.

At a perhaps more fundamental level, cultures affect the way in which researchers think about the world. There are some research questions being asked today which could not have even been thought of in previous eras. Some developments in current physics, for example, have been research programmes that seek to discover the origin of the universe, with various hypotheses such as the 'big bang' theory being proposed. That these questions are being asked at all is a phenomenon not just of scientific development, but of cultural change. In earlier times these questions would not have been asked, or at least not so widely, because the answer was already 'known' – the universe was created by God. It is only in an increasingly secular society which has moved away from formal religious doctrine that this 'knowledge' becomes regarded as questionable.

The 'hard' sciences therefore, are not as depersonalized as we would like to believe. What then of the 'soft' sciences, for example sociology? One way of describing the history of sociology, which admittedly runs the risk of crude oversimplification, is to say that it began by seeking to replicate the methods of the hard sciences. Thus we have Durkheim, often regarded as the founder of sociology, writing about 'social facts' in very much the way that a biologist or chemist would talk about scientific facts. In the early days of sociology as a recognized discipline, the view seems to have been that the social world could be regarded as roughly equivalent to the physical world, and that the same methods and approaches could be used to study both.

Whether this argument was based on genuine conviction, or whether it was made in order to achieve academic respectability, is a matter for the historians of sociology to debate. The result was a discipline which to us, now, looks strangely mechanistic and barren. There was a view of the researcher as a possible source of contamination, a concern with replication and methodological protocol, and an emphasis on objectivity. Sociology, in its early days, was a depersonalized science.

PERSONALIZED RESEARCH

This view of sociology was challenged in the 1930s by what became known as the Symbolic Interactionist school. Originating mainly from the work of Mead (1934), this group of sociologists began to see their subject matter – society – as fundamentally different from the subject matter of the life scientists. Mead argued that societies and the people in them do not have fixed properties which can be easily measured, but instead are constantly changing, not simply in response to external influences but because of their innate nature and abilities. The ability of people to communicate in symbols, and to negotiate meaning through their interactions with each other, meant that they could not be regarded simply as inert objects, but were dynamic and creative beings. The proper object of sociological study was therefore the creativity of people in their interactions with each other.

This change in the subject matter of sociology required some change in research methodology. If the focus of research was to be negotiation and interaction, then clearly this could not be studied by questionnaires or examination of demographic data. The researcher had to be able to witness and record these interactions. The solution that was developed was the method now known as participant observation: in other words, the researcher participated in the social world while observing it.

Participant observation is clearly very different from the distant and depersonalized methodology of early sociology. By participating in the world of the research subjects, the researcher ceases to be an anonymous figure and becomes an individual with particular attributes, which will shape the data as much as the attributes of those being studied. This change in approach to research led many orthodox sociologists at the time (and since) to criticize interactionist methodology for its subjectivity and consequent unverifiability. If data are partly the product of the researchers' interactions with research subjects, and these interactions are unique to the individual researcher, then they cannot be verified by replication by another researcher. As the interactions are so numerous, intangible and transient, they cannot even be documented with any degree of accuracy which would enable others to evaluate them.

The interactionists countered these criticisms in several ways. First, they argued that replication and generalization were not concerns of their research. They argued that because the research was conducted in unique contexts it was impossible to replicate anyway. They also argued that they were not trying, as sociologists had previously attempted, to develop 'laws' of human behaviour which could be generalized to other contexts: they were not trying to discover what would always happen, but what could happen.

These responses went some way to counter objections to their method, but there is a suggestion in their methodological writings that the interactionists had taken some of it to heart. Numerous research strategies are discussed in these texts which imply that the writers themselves had some concerns over the verifiability of data. Thus some texts exhort researchers to make copious detailed research notes or diaries, in order to document the interactions and processes that occur during field work. These are often portrayed as being for the benefit of the researcher, but could also be useful supportive evidence for any research conclusions in the face of criticism from others. Other writers, for example Denzin (1970), suggest 'triangulation' as a research strategy, in other words the use of multiple methods or settings or time periods to confirm or challenge interpretations. Triangulation seems something of an anomaly in interactionist research – a method used in geography to locate permanent physical features hardly sits well with the notions of dynamic and changing social life as it is described by the interactionists.

Despite the avowed rejection of 'objective' sociology, there is therefore some suggestion that the interactionists still retained some of its concerns, or at least did not feel that they could completely reject them and prosper as a respectable alternative. This concern over academic respectability partly centres on the notions of fact and truth evident in early sociology, but also on the idea that research should be something that only researchers can do – it should be more than journalism or anecdote. In other words, whereas anyone can tell a story about an event, there should be some difference between this story and the story told by a researcher – the researcher's story should display some difference in perspective or perception which can only be achieved through specialized study and training.

Thus whereas the interactionists sought to uncover the 'emic perspective' (in other words, the way in which research subjects saw their world) and placed great value in reproducing research subjects' own words, this was always interpreted and illuminated by the researcher's perspective and words. The researcher's perspective was largely taken for granted, whereas the subjects' was scrutinized and, for a school that had begun to see the researcher as more than a data-collecting automaton, there was a distinct lack of discussion about the researcher.

One of the effects of this taking the researcher for granted was perceived by later researchers to be an imbalance in power between researcher and subject. The superior power of the researcher was exercised in two ways. First, the final product of the research, the report, paper or book, was written by the researcher, often with no input from the research subjects. The researcher, rather than 'telling it like it is' was actually 'telling it like I see it'. Thus the outside world would be presented with a version of events which would not necessarily correspond with the research subjects' views. The researcher therefore had control over the way in which the subjects would be perceived by others. Secondly, at an interactional level, the researcher exercised power over subjects in the collection of data. Put simply, what would happen would be that the researcher would ask for (and usually get) information from research subjects, and would offer very little in return. The researcher would avoid expressing opinions, views, or even giving personal details, in order to avoid the 'danger' of prompting responses to questions.

Interactionist research, therefore, while moving some way from depersonalized social science, had not adequately addressed some of the interpersonal issues it had uncovered. While focusing on interaction and negotiation between research subjects, it had largely taken the researcher's interaction for granted. Thus later schools of social research and theory took as one of their main concerns, exactly this issue – the relationship between researcher and researched.

Perhaps the most prominent of these schools are the new-paradigm (Reason, 1988), feminist (Roberts, 1988) and action research perspectives (Winter, 1987), although there are others. They all pay attention to the research relationship, with particular concerns expressed over the dimensions of power inherent in such interaction. Typically they conceive the researcher–researched relationship as a cooperative partnership, with mutual exchanges of information and insights and shared control over the progress of the research.

This may address some of the issues involved in research relationships, and has produced many rich and illuminating studies, yet these research approaches – perhaps they can be called personalized research – still do not quite solve all the problems of the practitioner researcher. There is still an assumption that the researcher is to a great extent, an outsider. This is what makes mutual exchange of perspectives possible – there is a difference between perspectives. Feminist research does go some way towards recognizing shared experience in that it focuses on the issues affecting women, providing a common ground for researcher and researched, and drawing upon a well-established body of thought and theory about women's lives. If the study is not primarily about women's experiences, however, the theory that informs feminist research cannot be easily adapted to support it.

Perhaps the key to understanding the position of the practitioner in practitioner research, therefore, is to develop a theoretical basis analogous to feminist theory; in other words, a framework of concepts and notions about what it is to be a practitioner and what it means to do practitioner research. This book is an attempt to stimulate this development.

TOWARDS AN UNDERSTANDING OF
PRACTITIONER RESEARCH

The above discussion of research highlights two central themes in relation to the development of practitioner research. The first is the relationship between the researcher and the research subjects. The second is the relationship between the researcher and the data. The remainder of this chapter goes on to highlight distinctive aspects of practitioner research which arise from the differences in these relationships.

As discussed above, traditional social science approaches to research assume the researcher to be an 'outsider' or visitor to the research setting, whose sole purpose is to undertake research. Practitioners undertaking research into practice can, however, have a range of different relationships with the research setting, in terms of both role and knowledge. These relationships can perhaps best be explored along a continuum.

RESEARCHER POSITIONS

'OUTSIDER'	'HYBRID'	'INSIDER'
A researcher undertaking research into practice with no professional experience	A practitioner undertaking research into the practice of other practitioners	A practitioner undertaking research into their own and their colleagues practice

In the above continuum the 'outsider' position represents the traditional social science researcher undertaking research into the work of professional practitioners. Here, the researcher remains a visitor to the world of the practitioner throughout the research. The 'hybrid' role represents the practitioner undertaking research into the practice of other practitioners, for instance a nurse researcher undertaking research into nursing which is being carried out in a setting with which the nurse researcher is unfamiliar. This can be contrasted with the insider researcher, where a practitioner is undertaking research in their own workplace, into their own practice and the practice of their colleagues.

Using the notion of a continuum seems to us to be a flexible way of thinking about research positions, given that it is perfectly possible and probable that practitioner researchers will move backwards and forwards through a range of positions during the course of a study. For the purpose of our discussions, however, we have tended to illustrate our points by drawing upon examples from the extremes of the continuum, i.e. the complete outsider and the complete insider. Although we feel that this does enable us to present our arguments clearly, we are also aware that, as a result, we may have oversimplified the complexities of research positions and roles.

RESEARCH AIMS

For the social science researcher or 'outsider' the aim of the research is usually to contribute to the body of social science knowledge. Hence the research seeks to develop knowledge of social science concepts such as professionalization, socialization, cognitive dissonance or other concepts which are used to describe the ordering of the social world. Under these circumstances the research subjects, i.e. the practitioners, are only useful insofar as they contribute to the development of social science knowledge.

It is clear that a lot of the knowledge developed by social scientists is very useful to practitioners. Indeed, in recent years the social science curriculum has become a central component of most professional educational programmes. However, although concepts such as professionalization, socialization and behaviourism are very useful to practitioners, they do not meet the total needs of the practitioner in relation to practice knowledge.

This is particularly the case when the aims of social science research are contrasted with the aims of practitioner research. Under the traditional social science perspective the practitioner is both the subject and the user of research, but never the developer. As practitioners learn about the findings of social science research so they incorporate these into their practice. This then becomes the subject of further social science research. It is practitioners who remain under the microscope, rather than their practice. For the social scientist, therefore, practice is only examined for what it contributes to an understanding of practitioner action, not practitioner knowledge.

The aims of social science research can be contrasted with the aims of practitioner research. The primary aim of practitioner research is usually to solve a critical problem or to develop an understanding about the nature of practice, and ultimately to contribute to the body of professional knowledge. The distinction between social science knowledge and professional knowledge, although subtle, is important, as it indicates a different focus or concern. For instance, practitioner research is unlikely to be interested in developing knowledge about the concept of professionalization; what it might be interested in is understanding how the power relationship between the professional and the client can be altered in favour of the client, their relatives or an external agency advocating on their behalf. Alternatively, it might be interested in articulating tacit knowledge used by professionals during the course of their interaction with clients, and the impact of this tacit knowledge on power relationships.

Practitioner research, therefore, seems to be about improving practice. The introduction of the notion of *improvement* is critical to an understanding of practitioner research and, from a methodological perspective, possibly the most important distinguishing characteristic. Improvement of practice, and the expansion of the practitioner's knowledge base entailed in this endeavour, is an intrinsic motivator, determiner and aim of most forms of practitioner research. This aim is frequently translated into a simplistic but extrinsic objective. For instance, practitioner research might deliberately set out to identify the *most* comfortable position for a patient suffering from a particular condition, or the *best* method of emptying a urinary catheter bag. Issues such as these are unlikely to be addressed by social scientists as social science shies away from making judgemental statements. Traditionally social science has tended to view such statements as normative or culturally determined. From this perspective, judgemental statements are only interesting insofar as they inform the social scientist about underlying concepts, such as, in the above examples, 'comfort' or the 'social control of body products'. Social science research does not seek the *best* method for managing this aspect of social behaviour; rather, it seeks to understand the manifestation of these universal concepts in the context of nursing care as it has evolved within a particular cultural setting.

From the perspective of social science the use of value judgements (e.g. *best method*) as a yardstick for examining practice introduces, from the inception of the research, a culturally subjective bias which negates any claims to scientific rigour. This illustrates how the aims of practitioner research can be denied by the principles underpinning social science research. This arises from the methodological perspective developed in social science which negates the validity of value-laden research when it is judged against the criteria of academic rigour developed for the purposes of social science.

That social science is not primarily concerned with or able to recognize how to bring about improvements in care can be illustrated by a project set up in the early 1980s in the South East Thames Regional Health Authority. It was instigated by a charge nurse who had worked for some 30 years on a long-stay young disabled unit. Many of these patients were physically handicapped as a result of injuries sustained following accidents, including road traffic accidents. All of the patients had severe physical contractures of their limbs, which made them very deformed. The charge nurse became convinced that many of the patients were in extreme pain because their bodies were so misshapen that it was impossible to sit or lie them comfortably in conventionally shaped chairs and beds, which were all that was available. After many years' campaigning to raise interest in this issue, he managed to persuade a visiting dignitary to raise money via a charity to support a project to help with this problem. A student from the London School of Furniture was recruited who designed individual pieces of furniture shaped to the specific contours of each patient's misshapen body. The result was remarkable: patients who had writhed around for years, presumably in agony, although it was impossible to measure, became still and appeared comfortable. Some took to reading books for the first time in years, watching television, playing chess and generally communicating in ways that had been thought to be beyond their mental capacity for many years.

This type of project illustrates how practitioner research takes a very different theoretical stance towards issues of comfort or discomfort. In this case discomfort was taken for granted: the charge nurse felt no need to prove it – he'd witnessed it for 30 years and the point was to do something about it. Yet the very language within which research proposals are presented would require him to confirm what he already knew, in order to convince others that his insights were not subjective, which in fact they were. The difficulties involved in rendering the subjective objective for the purposes of research funding would probably militate against the funding of such a project even today. As a result the research would be unlikely to progress to the point of the project, which was doing something about the discomfort, rather than merely measuring it or theorizing about it.

It remains extremely difficult, even today, to get this kind of research funded. It is non-theoretical, individual pragmatic research. Some might even argue it is not research as it is traditionally recognized, although the person who designed the furniture was awarded a PhD for her work. The debate as to whether or not this is 'true' research in social science terms is irrelevant to the practitioner. It is clearly an avenue where massive *improvements* in practice could be made with very little recourse to formal theory. The lack of formal theory means that it might not be considered as formal research, but to argue this is to miss the point: that whether it is research or development, or whatever one wishes to label it, it requires funding, if only because of the immediate and massive decrease in human suffering it brought about for a relatively small amount of expenditure.

In this case no attempt was made to measure change, or indeed the ensuing improvements, except in the form of photographs, which gave to the viewer compelling evidence of improvement. The research was in the design of the furniture, which required an outsider specialist but an insider to see the need. Such an insider would not, as in this case, have the technical knowledge to put together a specialist proposal, neither would they necessarily have the contacts nor the status required to make such contacts, as again was very clear in this case.

The above example also illustrates how practitioner research is not only explicitly but also intrinsically about improving practice. It is about articulating and respecting the tacit knowledge of experienced practitioners. It is also about developing methods which enable us to recognize the importance of experience in contributing to practice and developing the knowledge base of practice. As well as the above example, which is a classic illustration of the use of tacit, experiential knowledge, two further examples of this approach to practitioner research are the work of Hunt (1991) and Lawler (1991). Both could be classified as hybrid practitioners on the above continuum, as both were qualified nurses, but their research into nursing was not directly into their own practice. Both researchers undertook a qualitative analysis of the knowledge developed by experienced practitioners in areas of practice that tend to be hidden from public scrutiny. Hunt looked at the ways in which experienced practitioners communicated with terminally ill patients, drawing extensively on examples of conversations recorded between nurses and such patients. Lawler looked at how experienced nurses managed the socially embarrassing situations encountered when patients are forced because of illness to perform private functions such as excreting, in front of nurses.

It is possible to argue that the work of both Hunt and Lawler is not strictly practitioner research, in that they did not undertake research directly into their own practice. Instead, they used qualitative research methods to articulate the knowledge used by practising nurses. As such, their work conforms closely to the tenets of new-paradigm research (Reason, 1988) and feminist research (Roberts, 1988). Both these methods advocate the development of a collaborative relationship between the researcher and the research subject; in both cases, however, the researcher remains an outsider, not only to the research setting but also to the practice knowledge. What distinguishes the work of Hunt and Lawler from new-paradigm or feminist research is their sharing of a common professional knowledge base, which informs not only their analysis of the data but also their awareness of issues worthy of research. Here insider knowledge is used not merely to collaborate with a social science project but, more importantly, to determine the project itself. Moreover, both projects set out to articulate the tacit knowledge developed by experienced nurses in order to *improve* the professional knowledge base of nursing.

Although feminist research, new-paradigm research and action research have many insights to offer the development of practitioner research, the crucial issue of control over aims will invariably be determined by the orientation of the researcher. Spendiff (1993) gave a particularly insightful account of this process in which she described some of the tensions that arose in her research when she used feminist methods while researching the experiences of women who described themselves as non-feminist. As Spendiff's paper clearly indicates, outsider researchers, whether they adopt progressive or traditional social science perspectives, are highly likely to be orientated to the social science agenda which arises out of the particular methodological stance they have adopted. This is partly because the researcher, as an outsider, will be unfamiliar with the issues and concerns of the practitioners. As Elbaz (1991) points out, however (and as illustrated in the example given above of the redesign of furniture), it is also because much of the agenda of research, from its inception through to its funding, tends to be set by the concerns of academia rather than practice.

Part of the problem arises because practitioner knowledge tends to deal with ambiguity. Practitioners have to learn how to work with imperfect knowledge: they cannot wait for the results of a piece of research before they act, they must act with what is available. Practitioner research, therefore, deals with ambiguity and messy contextual dependent problems. Often, as in the above example about redesigning furniture, practitioners cannot 'prove' what they know through experience: this has to be taken on trust. It follows, therefore, that practitioner research draws heavily on 'insider' knowledge and experience, which often cannot be articulated in ways that conform to traditional research proposals.

For practitioners, then, the aim of research, either implicitly or explicitly, is to improve practice with all the judgemental, normative agenda that this implies. Because of this agenda, practitioner research has an inbuilt inherent bias towards good practice, however this might be defined. To a social scientist such a starting point for research is heretical because all such notions of 'good' or 'improvement' are in themselves questionable and, by definition, problematic, i.e. what do we mean by *good*? or *improvement on what*? Although this may be the end point of research, it can never be the starting point.

There is, therefore, a subtle but important difference in the aims of social science research as against practitioner research. This difference is important because it influences the subsequent direction of the research at each stage in the process.

DESIGN AND PLANNING OF THE RESEARCH

Design is a crucial aspect of any research project; this is as true for qualitative research as it is for quantitative, more experimental approaches to research. In each case issues of sampling, questioning and observing dominate discussions about the design of the research. Virtually hundreds of research methods textbooks have been published offering advice to the researcher on how to tackle these complex issues. Surprisingly, few if any consider the position of the practitioner researcher. Most assume the researcher to be an outsider, or at least a hybrid, embarking on a research study into the practice of others and not directly into their own practice. This gives rise to a number of design and planning issues which, for the insider researcher, differ at crucial points from the advice given to the outsider.

Choice of a research setting

For the outsider or hybrid researcher, the choice of a research setting tends to be quite open and is primarily circumscribed by theoretical issues of sampling alongside practical considerations of cost or travel arrangements. An insider, on the other hand, may have little or no choice about any of these issues. Their research setting will be their place of practice. The primary reason for this is that they want to undertake research into an aspect of their own practice. It makes sense, therefore, to undertake the research in their own practice setting. The second reason is ease of access. It is often quite easy for practitioners to gain access to their own practice setting, but more difficult for them to gain access into another clinical area. This is partly because as a working practitioner they are not negotiating access from a 'neutral' academic environment, but from a practice-based setting. In the present climate of market forces, access into a competitor's clinical area for the purpose of research may be viewed with considerable suspicion.

Finally, if the researcher is an insider then they are simultaneously a working practitioner, and they therefore have to undertake the research alongside their role as a full or part-time clinician. This means that, at a practical level, they have very little spare time to give to the research. What time they have would be considerably reduced, by travelling time if nothing else, if the research was conducted in a range of different clinical settings. For these reasons, practitioner research frequently involves research undertaken in one's own clinical area or area of expertise.

Negotiation of role

Consequently, the insider practitioner researcher, unlike the outsider or hybrid researcher, may occupy a number of different roles simultaneously within the research environment. The outsider or hybrid researcher visits the research setting purely for the purposes of research, and therefore occupies the singular temporary role of researcher. The insider practitioner researcher, however, may also be a working colleague of those being researched. They may also be the person in charge of the unit and so the manager of the people being researched. Alternatively, they may be a subordinate member of staff and have to interview people who in different situations manage them. Invariably they are also peers of at least some of their research subjects.

The multiplicity of roles held by the practitioner researcher is extremely complicated and has to be taken into consideration in the design of the research. There is no point in designing a piece of practitioner research which depends on colleagues giving you information in your role as researcher that they would be unwilling to impart to you in other roles, as they are unlikely to be forthcoming. Although this might seem like a weakness it can be construed as a strength of insider practitioner research. First, it indicates a degree of insider knowledge about the unit that an outsider researcher would be unlikely to discover until well into the research programme. The starting point for insider research is, therefore, extremely well informed. The issue is how to use insider knowledge both constructively and ethically: constructively to inform the design of the research, and ethically to elicit the maximum amount of information within the multiplicity of roles held within the unit.

Secondly, it could be argued that the multiplicity of roles is a disadvantage to the insider researcher as it may prevent them from eliciting information that would be given to an outsider researcher, whose singular role means they do not pose a threat to the research subject. However, if the information is to be used by the outsider researcher they will need to make it public. One of the problems with in-depth qualitative studies is disguising the source of information. A research subject is therefore no more likely to reveal politically sensitive information to an outsider researcher than to an insider researcher. If they do, they may not wish it to be used, thus severely undermining its value.

Finally, it is important to remember that the insider practitioner researcher has a continuing relationship with research subjects that predates the research and which is likely to continue after the completion of the research. This makes it extremely difficult for the researcher to step in and out of role. It also raises questions about data access. Conversations over coffee, for instance, may provide crucial insights into the research question, or even conversations held in the past and resurrected as they appear to have a bearing on the research question. However, data such as these might not be considered legitimate, as the researcher was in the role of practitioner at the time of the conversation, and the person making the remark may not be happy to have it included in the research. Similarly, an action observed during the course of practice may provide evidence for the research, again making the distinction between the role of researcher and practitioner difficult to sustain. This issue can be partly addressed by asking permission to include the remark or observation in the research. However, this might further complicate the research setting as colleagues become aware that all remarks or nursing behaviours are a source of potential data whenever the practitioner researcher is on duty.

Such a situation may well interfere with other roles held by the researcher in the unit, such as supporter or manager. People might be reluctant to confide in the researcher as they might under normal circumstances, in case permission is then sought to use information gained in these circumstances in the research. In seeking support from the researcher a colleague might not want to appear unsupportive by subsequently refusing permission for their experiences to be used as research data. Research methods textbooks all address issues of informed consent and the contractual or collaborative arrangements between the researcher and the research subjects. They rarely, if ever, address issues of reciprocity and allegiance in research settings.

The above discussion about the negotiation of role appears to raise two issues in relation to insider practitioner research: the first is the politics of the situation and the second is the pragmatics of the situation. Although both issues are discussed extensively in research methods books, in particular feminist, new-paradigm and action research methodology textbooks, they tend to be discussed from the perspective of the outsider researcher.

Feminist, new-paradigm and action research all recognize and discuss the importance of the political context in which the research is taking place. They highlight issues such as how researchers should sensitize themselves to the politics of the organization and how such politically sensitive data should be written up. However, they tend to discuss these issues from the perspective of the outsider collaborative re-searcher. For an insider practitioner researcher this is only half the picture: they must also come to terms with the fact that, as a practi-tioner, they are crucially involved in the politics of the research setting, that they had some part to play in the creation of the political situation and in its continuation.

From a pragmatic perspective the insider practitioner researcher must also come to terms with the impact of the research on the clinical environment. This raises two main issues: the impact of the research on the therapeutic environment and the issue of reciprocity: in return for the cooperation of colleagues with the research, the researcher might have to barter or negotiate other aspects of their role and conform with demands made by colleagues over other issues within the unit.

Part of the problem seems to stem from the conceptualization of the researcher as a single individual, working under supervision but essen-tially in isolation. How true this is of modern-day research is a moot point. Few texts, or indeed academic institutions or funding bodies, seem able to deal with the concept of team research without frequent recourse to an identified team leader or principal investigator. For this reason alone, the insider researcher must isolate their research activities from their practitioner activities, as the idea of group research, rather than single projects, is difficult for many academic institutions to accom-modate and accredit.

From the research perspective, this severely limits the extent to which the insider practitioner researcher can intervene in the clinical environment to test out changes or improvements in practice. Unless they hold a senior or authoritative position within the organization it might be difficult for the single researcher to introduce a change in practice or set up an experiment to test out innovations in practice. This is partly because such changes necessarily require not only the agreement or consent of colleagues, but also their active cooperation. Such cooperation will have to be negotiated within the multiplicity of roles, and might require compromise by the researcher in other roles to accommodate colleagues' projects.

A special case – the clinical controlled trial

Even if it is possible to negotiate the introduction of an innovation for the purposes of research, the format of the research might interfere with or confound the perceived therapeutic aims of the unit. This is more likely to be the case if the researcher adopts a traditional quantitative or experimental approach to research, such as the clinical control trial. Here, the researcher might find that the allocation of clients to control groups conflicts with therapeutic aims derived from their role as practitioner. Two interesting examples of this dilemma are discussed later in the book. First, Chris Stevenson gives an interesting example of this problem in Chapter 6, where she describes how her attempts to produce a quantified evaluation of an aspect of her practice, namely family therapy, were at odds with the therapy itself, forcing clients to produce structured statements in the midst of a fluid, painful and ill-defined change process. The second example, by Val Pirie, described in Chapter 5, illustrates the problems of attempting to use the clinical control trial to test experimentally whether the use of hand puppets improves communication between nurse therapists and small children. The problems of adopting an experimental method when working with small children are graphically illustrated, as children cannot be expected to conform to the rigours of standardized experimental design.

Adherents of the clinical control trial, however, argue that it is by far the strongest method of clinical research, producing the most convincing evidence. Although adherents recognize ethical dilemmas in experimental clinical research, they argue that such dilemmas arise because the effect of the experiment on the research subject is unknown. They therefore seek to minimize risk to the research subjects. Adherents of the clinical control trial would deny, however, that a conflict can arise between the imperatives of the experiment and the imperatives of therapy, arguing that if the researcher perceives a therapeutic loss to a particular group, they have not understood the basic principle of controlled trials, which is to test the effectiveness of a given therapy.

Although this might be the case when testing a technological innovation such as a new drug, it is not necessarily the case when introducing a new practice, which is usually being advocated because earlier research has highlighted its effectiveness. For instance, practitioner research designed to improve the quality of information given to patients is based on earlier research which indicates the importance of patient knowledge in promoting compliance with therapeutic regimens. If a controlled trial is used to test the effectiveness of a particular method of improving patient information, one group of patients will not be subjected to the new method while an experimental group will be. In order to measure the effectiveness of the new regimen, however, the knowledge of both groups will be tested at regular intervals. If, during the course of testing, the practitioner researcher comes across a gross knowledge deficit on the part of one of the patients, their practitioner role would strongly incline them to correct this deficit. Indeed, not to do so could break the professional regulations or codes of conduct that they are subject to in their practitioner role. From an experimental perspective, however, correcting the knowledge deficit is tantamount to contaminating the experiment, as the knowledge deficit only came to light because of instruments used for research purposes to measure knowledge acquisition.

An outsider researcher, particularly a non-practitioner, is possibly in a better position to conduct such research, simply because they can claim ignorance of the possible impact of the knowledge deficit for the health of the patient. However, to make such a claim is a weak defence because clearly, solving the problem of ignorance by using a researcher whose own lack of knowledge renders them unable to detect ignorance is no defence at all. The issue needs to be tackled at the level of methodology and ethics. From this perspective action research, feminist research and new-paradigm research would all advocate that not only should the research do the subject no harm, but it should actively bestow benefits on them (Wilde, 1992).

Again we are back to the issue of improvement. Clinical control trials are about developing new knowledge, previously untested, where the benefits are not known in advance. Practitioner research is frequently about improvements – the benefits are therefore, by definition, known in advance, at least tacitly if not theoretically (see the example of furniture design given above). To argue against this is to argue against the generalization of knowledge and to suggest that every time knowledge is used it must first be tested for its efficacy in each environment in which it is applied. Such a suggestion is clearly absurd, and yet it frequently provides the criteria against which practitioner research proposals are judged.

More ominously, perhaps, demands are also frequently made to replicate studies prior to the implementation of the research-based knowledge in case 'it doesn't work here'. Such demands simply serve to prolong the process of implementation and indeed, if the research cannot be mounted, to prevent the dissemination of research findings.

DATA ANALYSIS

It is argued earlier in the chapter that qualitative research methods, and in particular the personalized methods advocated by feminist and new-paradigm research, are theoretically much more closely allied to practitioner research than traditional experimental or quantitative approaches to research. For this reason this section will concentrate on a discussion of the similarities and differences between qualitative data analysis and data analysis for practitioner research. This is because this is a grey area where methods have more in common than in difference. However, it is possible to discern subtle differences which will form the focus of the discussion.

Silverman (1985), in his discussion on qualitative research methodology, highlights a central concern for many qualitative researchers when he states that: 'The observer may "go native", identifying so much with the participants that, like a child learning to talk, he cannot remember how he found out or articulate the principles underlying what he is doing' (Silverman, 1985, p.105). This quotation highlights a central concern in social science research, which focuses on the relationship between the researcher and their data. For many qualitative social scientists 'going native', or identifying too closely with the participants in the research, introduces a subjective or partisan stance which undermines the validity of the analysis. Objective analysis, it is supposed, can only be obtained from adopting a disinterested involvement in the research. The roots of this perspective on data analysis can be traced back to the anthropological origins of sociology as a discipline. Indeed, Strauss and Corbin (1990), when discussing the analysis of qualitative data, emphasize the importance of rendering it anthropologically strange. They illustrate their argument with a discussion of a woman in a red dress in a restaurant. While her role as hostess might be obvious to someone familiar with the culture of restaurants, they suggest that this jumps too quickly from observation to culturally determined roles. It leaves out the important process of how roles come to be defined and maintained within a given culture. This intermediate level of analysis, Strauss and Corbin suggest, is the hallmark of good-quality qualitative sociological research.

The strength of this position is thought to reside in its ability to avoid the imposition of deductively determined categories of analysis on human behaviour. By rendering the data anthropologically strange, researchers avoid imposing their own categories of analysis (e.g. in the case of the woman in the red dress, hostess) on to the data. Instead, the analytical categories *emerge* from the data by an inductive process of categorization and comparison.

This process is well documented in the work of Glaser and Strauss (1967), who developed the idea of grounded theory as a method of qualitative data analysis. They were very concerned to avoid deductive processes of data analysis, to the extent that they advised against undertaking a literature review prior to the research, in case previously formulated theoretical frameworks interfered with the process of data analysis, thereby preventing the development of fresh insights or novel theoretical developments.

The adoption of this stance towards data analysis does, as Silverman (1985) points out, create considerable tension in qualitative research. Primarily it prevents the development of a body of cumulative theoretical knowledge, as each study is bound by both culture and context. Indeed, in an area such as nursing, where much of the work is routine, it might be possible to reinvent the wheel several times and never know it.

The work of Glaser and Strauss (1967) and Strauss and Corbin (1990) has, however, been particularly influential in nursing, and has formed the basis for a number of research studies. This does indicate that some problems might arise in the adoption of an anthropological stance towards practice, as practitioner researchers are, by virtue of their training, thoroughly socialized into the culture under study.

For this reason, developments in feminist research and new-paradigm research might be more helpful to us. Feminist research in particular recognizes the importance of taking a theoretical stand in relation to data. It argues the need for the researcher to declare their political position in relation to the data being collected. This means declaring aims not just in terms of knowledge development but also in terms of the moral worth of the research. If, as argued above, practitioner research is fundamentally about improving practice, this would seem sensible. It would require the researcher to identify not only earlier research evidence which suggests that the practice being advocated is an improvement, but also the moral basis for this. This can be illustrated by taking the example of the research into furniture adaptation again. The moral basis here was simple: a belief that pain could be reduced and comfort improved by more appropriately designed furniture. Although a theologically inclined researcher could discuss the edifying benefits of pain and put forward a case for maintaining it, most health care practitioners see the reduction of pain as an important aspect of their work and an area intrinsically worthy of further research.

However, once a position has been declared it then makes it very difficult for the researcher to argue that their data analysis was purely inductive. Clearly, the whole point of declaring a stand is to enable the reader to judge the subsequent analysis in the context of the stand taken. This, as Spendiff (1993) has highlighted, is a central tension in feminist research which, while recognizing the fallacy of rendering data anthropologically strange, has never quite identified other ways to validate the voice of the research subject independently from that of the all too powerful researcher.

In the tradition of feminist research we can offer our own version of how we think this tension may be addressed. We must emphasize that this is a personal perspective offered for the purpose of furthering the debate, rather than intending to solve the problem.

The issue of data analysis in qualitative research seems to turn on the use of theory. Traditional qualitative research has its roots in inductive theory-building approaches to data analysis. However, as the above discussion of feminist research indicates, it is necessary to distinguish between inductive theory generated from the researcher's interpretation of data and inductive theory which articulates the voice of the research subject. Bryman (1988) has discussed this tension in some detail and concludes that most qualitative research produces inductive theory that reflects the researcher's voice, rather than the voice of the research subjects. Indeed, Bryman agrees with Silverman (1985), both arguing that for qualitative research to do otherwise is to forfeit the responsibility of researcher and to do an inadequate job.

Feminist research, on the other hand, finds it more difficult to come down categorically on the side of the researcher. Feminist research recognizes that part of the problem with the research agenda in social sciences has been its failure to recognize the voice of oppressed sections of society, including women (Smith, 1988). Consequently, feminist researchers have consistently highlighted the importance of a democratic process of data analysis, which renders visible large areas of human experience that would remain untapped by social science research if it only recognized the interpretation of the researcher and not the researched. Feminist researchers, therefore, emphasize the dynamic interactive process of theory generation.

Both of these positions are helpful when thinking about practitioner research. It was argued above that practitioner research is distinguished by its primary aim, which is to improve practice, and that one method of doing this is to articulate the voice of the experienced practitioner and explicate the tacit knowledge that is embedded in practice. Such an approach turns on the use of theory. In traditional academic research, theory is the end point of all research and the starting point of quantitative research. Theory, however, can also be the product of research. As Silverman (1985) points out, it is also what demarcates research from other forms of writing: story-telling, novels and journalism. It is important, therefore, to discuss what is happening to theory in practitioner research.

If we consider the world of practitioner research, what we invariably discover is that theory is being used or implemented with a view to improving practice. This indicates that, like the feminist researcher, practitioner researchers must start by explaining why this theory is being implemented. What is good about it? Why do they suppose it will improve practice? To follow up the example used in the section on the clinical control trial above, why is improved communication considered to be intrinsically a 'good thing'?

It is necessary, then, to devise methods for data collection and to analyse the data collected from the perspective of the stated aim of the research, which was an improvement in practice. At this point it might be useful to consider a method of data analysis discussed by Silverman (1985), namely analytic induction. According to Silverman, analytic induction is a method of data analysis in which the qualitative researcher tries to formulate generalizations that hold across all the data collected. This is achieved by actively searching for negative cases. When one such case is found the researcher can either reformulate their theoretical framework to accommodate it or redraw the boundaries within which the theory can meaningfully apply. Silverman's account of analytic induction is particularly useful as he discusses the use of this method in relation to case study analysis, which is particularly pertinent for practitioner research. It can also be used with ethnographic and survey research, and been discussed in some detail by Denzin (1970) and Bulmer (1979).

The strength of this method for practitioner research, we would suggest, lies in its systematic search for negative cases. In other words, it instructs the researcher to search out data that do not fit the presuppositions of the research. In the case of practitioner research the researcher would attempt to collect data not to confirm that the implementation of theory, as expected, led to an improvement in practice, but which disconfirmed the initial assumptions of the researchers. In this way it is possible to highlight situations in which the expected improvements did not occur, and so to identify boundaries to the generalization of the theory into practice.

Such an approach is reminiscent of deductive theory testing, and therefore sits uneasily within a qualitative research framework. However, while it might be about testing theory, it is about testing theory qualitatively and not quantitatively – it is not about statistical significance, but about theoretical significance. Clearly, such research is very important in the arena of practitioner research, which starts out with an explicit aim of implementing existing knowledge in order to improve practice. It is important to identify those situations in which it does indeed do so and those situations where this is not the case. In so doing it is quite possible that fresh insights into practice will be generated, and that these will arise inductively from the dynamic tension created through the process of examining positive and negative cases.

The interesting aspect of this approach, when used in this way, is that practice and not theory becomes the end point of the analysis. Theory becomes a tool to explore the dimensions and boundaries of practice. This is in sharp contrast to traditional academic research, which uses practice to explore the dimensions of theory.

This proposition about using theory to explore practice, rather than the other way round, is radically different from the use of theory postulated in most research methods textbooks. This is possibly because for practitioner researchers the aim of the research is not an increase in the products of academia, i.e. theory, but an improvement in practice knowledge. It is also arguably what is actually happening in some of the most interesting recent research.

If we return to the work of Hunt (1991) and Lawler (1991), they both used well-established theoretical frameworks in the analysis of their data. Lawler's work drew heavily on anthropological literature on social taboos and body products. Hunt's work revisited theoretical perspectives on maintaining hope and motivation. However, neither researcher set out with the explicit aim of increasing theoretical knowledge about these concepts. If, during the course of their analysis this occurred, this was fortuitous, but not essential for the research. Instead, what both researchers sought to do was to identify how experienced practitioners dealt with these aspects of their work.

Although it is not possible to say for certain from reading the research, it appears that, although they used theory in very similar ways to inform the analysis of their data, Lawler's research was heavily influenced by her reading of the literature on social taboos and body products prior to data collection, which prompted her to be curious about how nurses, who clearly break these taboos every day, negotiate this delicate area. Hunt, on the other hand, did not appear to set out to look at the maintenance of hope or motivation at the start of her research: these themes arose from her analysis of the data. She was, however, able to use theoretical work already published in these areas as a method of categorizing and analysing her data.

Whatever the way in which the researchers arrived at their analysis, it is clear that it represents a tremendous step forward. In the past we have known about these issues from a theoretical perspective only. We could not, therefore, indicate how this knowledge could be used to inform practice in any direct sense. As with all social science research, the direct application of the findings was left to the user. For some it remained a blank page – mysterious, inexplicable and unexplained. As a result of the work of Lawler and of Hunt, 'meat' has been put on the 'bones' of these concepts. The use of these concepts in practice settings has been uncovered and revealed. It is possible that practitioners can now work in these areas with greater confidence, because their tacit knowledge has either been affirmed or informed by the research. Even if it contradicts the tacit knowledge of the practitioner this does not negate either the research or the practitioners' experience – it simply provides the starting point for further research into the subject.

The above discussion has examined the use of theory in practitioner research and argued that the debate about power and control over theory generation, which has dominated discussions of qualitative data analysis in the social sciences, ceases to be such a central issue in practitioner research. This is because the aim of practitioner research is not the generation of theory, and therefore ownership of theory is not a crucial indicator of academic output.

Instead, it is argued that the aim of practitioner research is the generation of practitioner knowledge. Theory is merely a tool that facilitates an unlocking of this knowledge. Under these circumstances, there is no particular need to claim an allegiance to either a deductive or an inductive approach to research. Indeed, an allegiance to improving practice takes precedence over this debate. Using the notion of analytic induction, theory can be used deductively or inductively: deductively in order to test out the applicability of theory to a given area of practice, or inductively in order to identify boundaries to the application of knowledge or situations which do not conform to the assumptions underlying the theory. Theory can also be used to facilitate the *post hoc* analysis of qualitative data, as demonstrated by Hunt. This approach is arguably very powerful, as it facilitates a much greater understanding of theoretical concepts that usually remain singularly abstract and hidden from public scrutiny.

DISSEMINATION AND COMMITMENT

The final stage of the research process is the dissemination of the findings. In traditional social science research, conducted by an outsider researcher, dissemination is invariably to the academic community whence the researcher came and to where they will return. Consequently, their primary commitment is not to practice but to the academic community, if for no other reason than that is where their future career lies.

Traditional social science researchers may, if time and funding permit (although they usually do not), feed back the results of the research to the participants. This can take the form of a presentation or a written report. Occasionally, if the findings are particularly relevant to an area of clinical practice they may be submitted to a professional journal as well as a social science journal, as a means of disseminating knowledge to practitioners.

Again, feminist and new-paradigm research have gone much further down the road of dissemination than traditional social science research. Both methods are concerned to democratize the research process. Good practice, using these methods, dictates a cyclical process of data analysis which actively involves the research participants. At the end of the research, the participants should have become so involved with the research process that they feel some ownership of the findings. Indeed, they may even be encouraged by the researcher to publish the results themselves in professional and/or social science journals.

During the course of this process it is inevitable that ethical issues will arise in relation to the publication of certain aspects of the findings. Some of the data may relate to politically sensitive issues, while other aspects may be damaging to the unit or indicate an area of poor practice that some of the research subjects would prefer not to be made public. These issues will have been hotly debated during the cyclical process of data analysis. A particular strength of this approach is that it gives the research subjects an opportunity to justify or rationalize their behaviour as the analysis progresses, and to give or withhold consent from an informed perspective. This is a much more sensitive approach than traditional social science research which, without the cyclical process of data analysis, could inadvertently betray the trust of the research subjects by revealing politically sensitive material in a clumsy or ill-informed manner.

The issue of dissemination and commitment is much more complicated, however, in insider practitioner research. Here the researcher has a commitment not just to the academic community, nor simply the professional community, but also to colleagues who took part in the research. All of these interests have to be balanced against each other in the analysis of the data and the dissemination of the findings.

As a result, both the analysis of data and the publication of findings may be circumscribed to accommodate the sensibilities of colleagues. Some might argue that accepting these limitations on the dissemination of the findings results in 'weak' research. Interestingly, this can be countered by adopting a committed stance towards *improving* practice, from the outset of the research. Adopting a committed stance in this case means emphasizing the positive, rather than the negative, aspects of practice. This might appear methodologically unsound; however, this is possibly only the case when looked at from the purist perspective of social science, which treats practice as a subject rather than an object of research.

If practice is treated as a subject of research, then it is important to capture and analyse all elements of that practice, regardless of the consequences for the research subjects. Alternatively, if practice is treated as an object (in the sense of an objective or aim) of research, where the central concern is to improve practice, then it is important that research explicitly sets out to focus on the circumstances and contexts that give rise to these improvements. The argument is not about ignoring or covering up negative aspects of practice; rather it is about focusing on positive developments and highlighting innovative practice in order to discover how we can remedy some of the negative aspects with which we are all too familiar.

Traditional approaches to social science are unable to fully develop this type of enquiry because of their overriding concern with authenticity. This prevents researchers from focusing on issues of improvement or innovation, as by definition such developments are not representative of the totality of the practice under consideration. As in quantitative research, the concern, in qualitative research, to capture all the elements of practice results in an averaging of the findings where positive aspects of practice are cancelled out by negative aspects. This prevents the development of a focused study of either positive or negative practices in their own right. This topic is worthy of further debate and consideration.

More importantly, perhaps, the strength of practitioner research lies in the integration of research with practice. With the exception of action research, traditional academic approaches to research have tended to disown the problem of implementation. This has been left to the professionals or practitioners and has rarely been viewed as the responsibility of the academics. The result of this dislocation between academia and practice is the development of a wide gap between theory and practice. This has been of some concern in nursing for a long time. It is increasingly a concern shared by other professions, who are experiencing similar difficulties in developing research-based practice.

A particular strength of practitioner research is the fact that from its inception it bridges this gap. The research process will almost certainly be influential on the development of practice within the unit, while the continued employment of the practitioner researcher at the end of the research ensures at least some continuity between findings and practice.

Practitioner researchers are, therefore, crucially concerned about how their findings are used. This is a much bigger issue than for outsider researchers, who may never encounter their research subjects again. Given the difficulties currently experienced in implementing research-based practice, this level of commitment and concern about how the research findings are used must be one of the core strengths of practitioner research.

CONCLUSION

In this chapter we have tried to introduce some of the ideas that underpin the notion of the practitioner researcher, i.e. practitioners who are researching their practice. These are not simply ideas about how the practitioner researcher is disadvantaged in relation to the traditional academic researcher in terms of their lack of distance or objectivity, but of how these characteristics might equally well be constructed as advantages for this particular kind of research. Figure 1.1 gives a summary of the main differences between methodological issues as they arise for traditional academic researchers and for practitioner researchers. Although it is probably verging on the polemic it provides a useful summary of the issues discussed in the latter half of this chapter. These differences lie in the person of the researcher, in their knowledge and goals, and we have argued that it is only relatively recently that such personal characteristics have been acknowledged in traditional research. If we begin to think about research as a personalized activity, then these characteristics have profound implications for the conduct of research studies.

The knowledge and goals of the practitioner researcher have been only briefly discussed here, but they are expanded upon in Chapter 2, which examines practitioner knowledge in more detail, and Chapter 3, which discusses the aims and objectives of practitioner research in more depth. What we have done, however, is to attempt to develop a set of criteria for conducting and evaluating practitioner research which reflects the particular nature of this type of enquiry. These criteria, however, will not fit all research done by practitioners, because some will prefer or wish to take a more traditional path, and there is a great deal to be said for multiple perspectives and approaches on issues as important as health care – we are not discounting the usefulness of health care practitioners leaving their current work, say through secondment, to work on research projects. We also accept that some people will seek to study topics of interest across regions or in unfamiliar settings, say through part-time courses which give them opportunities to learn a range of research methods, or to extend their knowledge in ways that would be difficult within the limitations of their own work environments. Some may even wish to train as professional researchers with a view to leaving direct employment in health care. However, such individuals have a large and diverse range of excellent methodology texts to choose from. This book is dedicated to those practitioners who wish to undertake research into their own practice, and therefore focuses and concentrates on their needs.

For those who use traditional approaches, the criteria we set forth here are not necessarily appropriate: traditional criteria are more relevant. By the same token, however, traditional research evaluation is not the best way to examine practitioner research. These debates about evaluation and criteria are extremely important to the development of practitioner research, and not simply as a defence against critics. By looking at the hallmarks of strong practitioner research, we can come closer to understanding, expressing and articulating what it is about, and what it can offer health care.

'OUTSIDER'	'INSIDER'
AIMS The primary aim of social science research is to explore a social phenomenon (nursing) in order to contribute to the body of social science knowledge	**AIMS** The primary aim of nursing research is usually to solve a critical problem, thereby contributing to the body of nursing knowledge
ACCESS The choice of a research setting is wide, but their contact is superficial	**ACCESS** Their choice of a research setting is limited but their contact is deep
NEGOTIATION OF ROLE The social science researcher is a *guest* in the world of nursing. They have a single role which is temporary	**NEGOTIATION OF ROLE** The nurse researcher is a *member* of the world being researched. They may have multiple roles, some of which are permanent
DESIGN & PLANNING Informed by knowledge of research methods	**DESIGN & PLANNING** Informed by insider knowledge and frequently governed by therapeutic imperatives
ANALYSIS Does not share taken-for-granted assumptions and is therefore able to adopt a naive stance towards the data	**ANALYSIS** Shares taken-for-granted assumptions the significance of which may not be recognized
DISSEMINATION & COMMITMENT To academic community to further academic knowledge. Not concerned about the everyday use of the research	**DISSEMINATION & COMMITMENT** To colleagues, professional and academic communities. Concerned about the way in which the research is used both locally and professionally

Fig. 1.1   Main differences between methodological positions.

REFERENCES

Bryman, A. (1988) *Quantity and Quality in Social Research*, Sage, London.
Bulmer, M. (1979) Concepts in the analysis of qualitative data. *Sociological Review*, **27**(4), 651–677.
Denzin, N. K. (1970) *The Research Act in Sociology*, Butterworths, London.
Elbaz, F. (1991) Research on teachers' knowledge: the evolution of a discourse. *Journal of Curriculum Studies*, **23**(1), 1–19.
Glaser, B. G. and Strauss, A. L. (1967) *The Discovery of Grounded Theory*, Aldine, Chicago.
Hunt, M. (1991) Being friendly and informal: reflected in nurses', terminally ill patients' and relatives' conversations at home. *Journal of Advanced Nursing*, **16**, 101–110.
Lawler, J. (1991) *Behind the Screens: Nursing, Somology and the Problem of the Body*, Churchill Livingstone, Edinburgh.
Mead, G.H. (1934) *Mind, Self and Society*, (ed. C. Morris), Chicago University Press, Chicago.
Reason, P. (1988) *Human Inquiry in Action: Developments in New Paradigm Research*, Sage, London.
Roberts, H. (1988) *Doing Feminist Research*, Allen and Unwin, London.
Silverman, D. (1985) *Qualitative Methodology and Sociology*, Gower, Aldershot.
Smith, D. (1988) *The Everyday World as Problematic*, Gower, Aldershot.
Spendiff, A. (1993) *Whose Reality? Feminist Research and Theorising with Non-Feminist Women*, Women's Studies Network (UK) Association Annual Conference, Nene College, Northampton 16–18 July.
Strauss, A. and Corbin, J. (1990) *Basics of Qualitative Research*, Sage, London.
Wilde, V. (1992) Controversial hypothesis on the relationship between researcher and informant in qualitative research. *Journal of Advanced Nursing*, **17**(2), 234–242.
Winter, R. (1987) *Action-Research and the Nature of Social Inquiry: Professional Innovation and Educational Work*, Avebury, Aldershot.

CHAPTER 2

The nature of practitioner knowledge

Liz Meerabeau

INTRODUCTION

Before going on to discuss the ways in which practitioner research may be developed, it seems useful to take some time in debating the type of knowledge that is the basis of such research. Practitioner knowledge informs research by guiding choice about research questions and research strategies, and a clearer understanding of what practitioner knowledge is (or, more accurately, what people have thought that it is) is a useful starting point.

This chapter aims to explore the concepts of tacit knowledge, reflective practice and experiential learning, drawing on literature from a variety of sources, including education and business studies as well as health care practice. Many of the issues involved in practitioner knowledge are common to several disciplines and reflect underlying changes in the philosophy of science as to what counts as legitimate knowledge; there have been changes both in the research methods used and the sorts of topics studied. The positivist tradition, however, still persists and has been prominent in the development of expert systems, or computer systems that mimic decision making, particularly in medicine (Caves, 1988; Jones, 1989).

The interactionist approach, however, views practitioner knowledge as messier but also involving more artistry. One of the themes of the literature discussed here is the reclamation of practitioner knowledge and the recognition that it is not just an inferior version of research-based knowledge (Benner, 1984; Carr and Kemmis, 1986; Schon, 1987); a corollary of this is that 'applying' knowledge is not as simple as it first appears. Since much interactionist work looks at how actors define their own situation, it may not be surprising that many of the concepts used in this chapter do not have precise definitions, or that different writers use them in rather different ways. Rather than getting bogged down in definitions, I prefer to explore the general ideas they put forward.

TACIT KNOWLEDGE

Berger and Luckmann (1967) consider that we are all unable to articulate knowledge which has become deeply sedimented, due either to our primary socialization as members of a society, or tertiary socialization as members of an occupational culture. To try to analyse our assumptions is like 'trying to push the bus in which we are riding'. Much of the literature on tacit, or unspoken, knowledge concerns expert practitioners. For example, Dreyfus (1981) argues that expert practitioners view situations holistically and draw on past concrete experience, whereas the merely competent or proficient must use conscious problem solving. Bhaskar and Simon (1977) claim that experts use economical, forward-looking strategies, whereas novices work backwards or use general strategies. For the expert, knowledge is embedded in their practice and is what Polanyi (1958, 1967) termed tacit knowledge. Tacit knowing is when we know something only by relying on our awareness of it for attending to a second activity; it is a hallmark of skilled practice, but also a feature of many everyday activities. Polanyi gives examples based on psychomotor skills, such as the coordination of respiration necessary to swim, or the action of hammering a nail, and also the useful example of recognising a friend's face, which we do without being aware of making comparisons with any other face. Not only are we unable to describe these skills but attention to the parts makes us unable to perform the whole. Polanyi (1958) also discusses scientific knowledge at some length. Again, practitioners draw heavily on tacit knowledge; they are unable to state their presuppositions and when they try they sound quite unconvincing: 'In effect, to the extent to which our intelligence falls short of the ideal of precise formalization, we act and see by the light of unspecifiable knowledge' (Polanyi, 1958).

Other philosophers and sociologists of science have discussed similar issues, for example Collins' (1974) study of work on lasers found that success always depended on personal contact between scientists; only then could they communicate the tacit, informal knowledge of how to build the laser. More recently, the controversy over cold fusion and its lack of replication was initially explained by assuming that Fleischmann and Pons, the chemists involved, had skills which their colleagues did not share (Close, 1991). The process of discovery is also thought to involve non-rational thinking. Kaufmann (1980) states that major discoveries involve a revealing 'flash of insight', and a switch from language to imagery. Koestler (1989) claims that discovery involves making novel links in the unconscious between previously unrelated concepts. Dreistadt (1968) states that scientists often use analogies and metaphors in making their discoveries; a famous example was Kekule, who discovered the cyclic structure of benzene and the aromatic hydrocarbons while daydreaming about snakes. These examples are important, since they indicate that, contrary to the popular view of science as a cerebral activity, it involves both creativity and considerable psychomotor skills.

Eraut (1985) also discusses practitioner knowledge, but relates it specifically to teaching. He begins by considering different kinds of professional knowledge, for example Oakeshott's (1962) distinction between technical knowledge, which can be written, and practical knowledge, which is similar to Polanyi's tacit knowledge, being expressed only in practice and learned through experience. Carr and Kemmis (1986) describe a range of teacher knowledge, from that which has its roots buried underground in practice, such as folk wisdom (students are restless on windy days; they are difficult on Friday afternoons), to that which has its 'head in the clouds of talk' such as educational theory, which must be made real and concrete to be understood. Broudy, Smith and Burnett (1964), looking at how knowledge is used, distinguish four modes: replication, application, interpretation and association. Replication dominates much of our initial education, whereas application involves the use of knowledge in new situations, although still by following rules. Eraut (1982) doubts whether in teaching it is possible to apply knowledge in any simple way, particularly the social sciences; at the most it provides a background understanding. Professional education involves the interpretation of knowledge, and provides ways of seeing a situation, although it may be difficult to break free and see situations in new ways. Particularly in a field such as education, interpretation may be idiosyncratic, or specific to a particular person or small professional group, since it involves an interplay between theory and practice. This is not surprising, since many situations in teaching depend heavily upon a particular context, and many of the concepts involved, such as pupil-centred learning, depend on the teacher fleshing out a concept or, to use a phrase from Macleod (1990), 'colouring it in'. Not only does an idea get reinterpreted, but it may need to be used before it acquires significant meaning. In putting an innovation into practice, we clarify our ideas in the process of implementation. Lastly, professional judgement may also involve intuition, or what Broudy, Smith and Burnett (1964) term association. This again resembles Polanyi's tacit knowledge, and often involves metaphors or images. Eraut (1982, 1985) also looks at the way in which knowledge is used. For example, the way that knowledge is used by an academic, who may wish to explore its problematic nature, will be different from the way it is used by the practising professional, who as a pragmatist wishes to find some sort of pointer for practice. The practitioner also has to develop routines and decision habits in order to keep mental effort to a reasonable level and avoid information overload. As Freidson (1971) states in his discussion of medical practice, the practitioner cannot suspend action in the absence of convincing evidence, nor afford to be sceptical, but often has to think on his or her feet. It thus seems inevitable that the researcher and the practitioner will use research-based knowledge in different ways.

In a later work, Freidson (1986) argues that much medical knowledge is neither formal and rational nor everyday common sense; it is specialist but non-formal; much of it is passed on by word of mouth. Eraut (1982) cites a similar finding from Farmer on orthopaedic surgeons, who have a detailed understanding of the stresses on bones but cannot express this in a formal engineering vocabulary. Also writing in the field of medical sociology, Jamous and Peloille (1970) and Atkinson, Reid and Sheldrake (1977) argue that tacit knowledge may be a positive asset, and is in fact the hallmark of a profession; they use the concepts of indeterminacy and technicality. Technicality refers to procedures that can be mastered and communicated in the form of rules, following a logical sequence as part of an efficient system. It has its roots in behaviourism, and concentrates on visible, observable performance, the sort which can be captured in expert systems. Indeterminacy refers to a variety of tacit and private knowledge which cannot be made wholly explicit; this model of 'professional artistry' stresses understanding, and takes a holistic approach. Many aspects of a profession can therefore be taught only through experience and close association with expert practitioners, and this can be used to draw occupational boundaries and limit access to the profession (although this strategy has its dangers, as we are now seeing in the skills mix debate).

These writers have examined several disciplines; Polanyi (1958) discusses a wide range of sciences. Eraut (1982, 1985) explores school teaching, and Freidson (1971, 1986), Jamous and Peloille (1970) and Atkinson, Reid and Sheldrake (1977) examine medicine. The consensus is that expert performance requires extensive, specific knowledge, which takes a long time to acquire but gives access to more powerful problem-solving techniques (Isenberg, 1991), and practitioners' knowledge is a sprawling and largely untapped resource. Research has been too narrowly defined by the academic community, who question why practitioners do not use research-based knowledge. If a broader framework is used, it is seen that practitioners do not merely 'apply' theory, but also create new knowledge, but it is often not codified or published, nor are reflection and discussion in the work environment easy. As Eraut (1985) states, 'Practical knowledge is never tidy, an appropriate language for handling much of it has yet to be developed.'

INTUITION

Several eminent writers on business and management have also addressed similar issues, under the rubric of intuition. For example, Agor (1989) argues that intuition is particularly useful in situations where there is a high level of uncertainty, where time is limited and there is a pressure to be right, and where there is little information, or the information does not favour one option over another. Isenberg (1991) states that managers often 'know' what is right before they can analyse it: they frequently act first and think later. What may appear as action for action's sake, however, is the result of intuitive under-standing that analysis is only possible in the light of experience gained while trying to solve the problem, since action is part of defining the problem. Mintzberg (1991) poses the question of why some brilliant management scientists cannot handle organizational politics, or why none of the techniques of business planning and analysis have had much effect on how top managers function, and answers his own questions by drawing on Ornstein's (1975) work on the left and right brain. Ornstein argues that analytical people such as accountants have better-developed left-hemisphere thinking processes, whereas artists and perhaps politicians have better-developed right-hemisphere pro-cesses. The two types of consciousness may be described as explicit versus implicit, verbal versus spatial, intellectual versus intuitive, or analytic versus gestalt. The first are privileged in western cultures and have been extensively studied, but we know little about the second; Berman (1990) says that western academic knowledge assumes that the body has nothing to tell us. Particularly at the higher levels of an organization, however, effective managers seem to revel in ambiguity and in mysterious systems with little apparent order; Mintzberg's own studies of senior managers have shown that key managerial processes draw on the vaguest of information and the least articulated of mental processes. A great deal of the managers' inputs are 'soft' and speculative, and managers prefer what they call 'the big picture', or a holistic approach. Mintzberg quotes the old story of the blind men trying to identify an elephant to illustrate that each person makes their own limited assessment, but the overall perspective is far more than the sum of these; he criticizes business schools for their overreliance on analytical techniques, and argues for a balance between these and skill-development techniques such as experiential learning.

HEALTH CARE PRACTITIONER KNOWLEDGE

The 'big picture' is also being explored in health care practice, particularly in nursing. Other health care professions are also debating these issues, but the discussion here will concentrate on nursing, mainly because of the extent of the published work which directly addresses practitioner knowledge. Benner (1984), for example, draws on work by Dreyfus and Dreyfus and Polanyi (1958) to gather accounts of what experienced nurses learn from their clinical practice. Further literature on nursing includes Vaughan (1992), who explores the nature of nursing knowledge, again drawing on the concept of tacit knowledge, and outlines three prime sources of knowledge: tenacity, expertise or authority, and logic. Carper (1978) has derived a frequently cited taxonomy of nursing knowledge in which there are four fundamental ways of knowing. These are empirics, in which knowledge is derived from observation (the positivist approach to knowledge), ethics, or moral knowledge, aesthetics or the art of nursing, and personal knowledge, or insight into how we ourselves function.

Younger (1990) argues that practitioner knowledge may also be developed by the use of literature. Vicarious experience can bridge gaps in the personal experience of the practitioner, and give 'the experience of life without its costs'. For example, the children's story *Charlotte's Web* (White, 1952) can be used to illuminate the meaning of caring. Ash (1992) uses photographs in a wide range of professional education settings; their ambiguity means that there are no 'right answers', and they summon up knowledge which is personal to the individual. Music and dance are less often used, Ash (1992) comments, because they are seen as 'decidedly non-academic and suspect'. Practitioner knowledge therefore ranges from the intuitive knowing of the experienced practitioner to research-derived knowledge. Both art and science are complementary. Rew and Barrow (1987), however, state that intuition is a neglected aspect of practitioner knowledge, and has only recently been recognized as a legitimate way of knowing.

REFLECTIVE PRACTICE

Schon (1987) also states that professional education neglects such knowledge and gives privileged status to systematic, preferably 'scientific' knowledge, which is often of marginal relevance to practice. He discusses 'knowing in action' (the sort of know-how we demonstrate in, for example, riding a bike) and 'reflection in action'. Usually, the latter occurs when our knowing in action does not go entirely to plan, but the two are not that distinct, and the expert probably uses reflection in action almost routinely. Like Jamous and Peloille, Schon recognizes both technicality and indeterminacy (although he does not use these labels).

Some professional work involves the routine application of facts, rules and protocols, such as the diagnostic procedure, but as the practitioner becomes more expert professional artistry becomes increasingly important. Although educators recognize that some practitioners have a particular expertise, good practice tends not to be a topic of enquiry. Taking the specific example of the business school, Schon discusses Simon's (1969) finding that there was a potential schism between the discipline-oriented and the profession oriented among those who taught business studies. Whereas Simon's solution was to make business studies more 'scientific', Schon, like Mintzberg, argues that: 'We should start not by asking how to make better use of research-based knowledge but by asking what we can learn from a careful examination of artistry' (Schon, 1987). To this end, Schon advocates the 'practicum', an intensive period of 'reflection in action' and reflection upon that reflection. Schon applies the concept of coaching to the highly skilled individual performances of the architectural studio and the conservatoire, but argues that it is a useful concept for any kind of professional education. He outlines three models of coaching: 'follow me', in which the student imitates the coach, joint experimentation, and hall of mirrors, in which both coach and student are involved in reflection upon the process of learning.

EXPERIENTIAL LEARNING

Boud (1989) claims that this is the most pervasive form of learning, but that it is devalued by educationalists because it is not abstract but rather practical and applied. Macleod (1990) examines how nurses learn from experience, by interviewing and observing ten 'expert' surgical ward sisters (quotation marks are used because the sisters, unlike their American counterparts, felt embarrassed by the label; Macleod attributes this to Scottish modesty). Macleod discusses the literature on experiential learning in some detail, including Kolb's (1984) cycle of learning; she concludes that the models used 'are grounded in experience, but do not excavate that ground'. Many do not really discuss the meaning of experience, tend to separate learning and reflection, and ignore the embodiment of knowledge.

This is a particular issue for Macleod, who remarks that clinical skills and knowledge are neglected in, for example, the studies of ward sisters, and that higher education courses for experienced nurses rarely enhance clinical know-how. She also wonders whether practical knowledge has been neglected in nursing because it recalls the past, when nurses knew only how and not why. It is a basic ploy of reformers to present the past in the least flattering light and we may have neglected the benefits of 'sitting next to Nelly', who may have been an expert in her own way.

Macleod's approach, based on Heidegger's hermeneutic phenomenology, looks at a personal world which cannot be separated from the self. Both the speaker and the listener contribute to meaning (the hermeneutic circle), and it is recognized that the interpretation given is not the only one. Unlike Benner (1984), Macleod found few well-formed narratives, although all the sisters had stories and 'watershed' experiences, which were often emotionally charged and led to changes in understanding. They also had resonant experiences, but the majority was taken-for-granted experience, or 'bits and bobs'. Learning was by a mix of acting, understanding and noticing, including the use of all the senses, highlighting the importance of embodiment. Macleod, like Ash (1992) and Benner (1984), also stresses the importance of the practitioner's engagement with practice; they cannot be a disinterested observer.

Embodiment is a growing area of study in sociology (Turner, 1992). It is also an important issue for Lawler (1991), who argues that the organization of what counts as legitimate knowledge prevents a comprehensive understanding of embodied experience, since knowledge is divided between different disciplines and much practitioner knowledge about how to manage the body is unofficial. The civilizing process (Elias, 1978) has privatized the body and barred it from 'normal' social discourse. Health care practitioners have an understanding of the body and of human existence which is fundamental to their practice, but this knowledge is not well documented and has not counted as 'proper' knowledge. Lawler claims that nursing is marginalized, not only because of its problematic knowledge base but because it is a largely female occupation. This brings us full circle, since part of the shift in the understanding of nursing knowledge and, in the human sciences more generally, has been the debate on 'malestream' knowledge and whether the ways of knowing discussed in this paper constitute a female perspective (Harding, 1991).

IMPLICATIONS FOR RESEARCH

The debates outlined above represent the work of writers and researchers who have attempted to explore the nature of practitioner knowledge. Their ideas and findings are by no means definitive; rather they represent some ideas about how we can start to conceptualize such knowledge. It is clear, however, that there is much more to be done in order to learn more about what we know and how we know it, and there are some indications about how we should proceed with this endeavour.

One such indication is that we should be wary of research into practice which relies entirely upon reports of that practice as a proxy for observation (Becker and Geer, 1957). Several studies (e.g. Fielding, 1986) have examined the perceived discrepancies between student nurses' espoused theories and their theories in use, to employ a distinction drawn by Argyris and Schon (1974), who point out that we are rarely able to give an accurate commentary upon our activities. Lincoln and Guba (1985) also recognize that we are liable to reinterpret our experience: 'Rationalizing...is nothing more than sense making in the face of chaos, subconscious behaviour, tacit knowledge, and outright forgetfulness. It is part and parcel of reality construction for individuals and institutions to engage in *ex post facto* reasoning to justify, explain, attribute, or make sense of behaviour.'

Both Lawler (1991) and Macleod (1990) observed participants in the work setting and then interviewed them about their perceptions of the observed events, as did Smith (1992). Lawler argues that this requires an 'insider' to appreciate the nuances of what is being discussed, although paradoxically tacit knowledge may also mean that there are many features of our practice which may require an outsider to research, since we are unable to make them 'anthropologically strange' (Dingwall, 1977). It is, of course one of the perennial concerns of the anthropologist that if they stay too long in one setting they may acquire tacit knowledge of the society, and therefore 'go native' and be unable to continue their analysis of the culture. A further objection which is sometimes raised to insider research is that it is 'biased', but this objection of course implies that it is possible to do 'neutral' research from a value-free position (Carr and Kemmis, 1986). The implication therefore seems to be that, wherever possible, research into practice should involve observation of that practice.

Observational research has its own problems, however. It takes place in real time and is therefore expensive and small-scale; it can also be stressful for both researcher and researched. The problem of an 'observer effect', though often anticipated, does not seem to be a difficulty in the hospital setting, where both staff and patients seem to adjust fairly rapidly to the presence of a researcher (Emerson, 1963). In community care it is more difficult, since the patient–practitioner dyad becomes a triad (Kratz, 1978). An alternative may be to use audio recording, as Fielding (1986) did in the hospital setting. It is not clear what method Schon (1987) used in obtaining his data, although their detailed quality implies either participant observation or audio recording; Benner (1984) used interviews, although they were of an unstructured kind. Much of her material, however, concerns fairly dramatic events in critical care settings, and it has proved difficult to use her approach in the less dramatic setting of care of the elderly, where arguably the need for this kind of work is all the greater (Reed, 1994). Benner comments that expertise can only be captured by qualitative context-dependent methods. As Miles (1979) observes, however: 'Qualitative data tend to overload the researcher badly at every point: the sheer range of phenomena to be observed, the recorded volume of notes, the time required for write up, coding, and analysis can all become overwhelming'. For Miles, qualitative data is an 'attractive nuisance' with few guidelines for its analysis, although this is now improving with the publication of qualitative methodology texts (e.g. Chenitz and Swanson, 1986) and the development of computer programs (Fielding and Lee, 1991). Ironically, the research methods have themselves had a large component of tacit knowledge.

Practitioner knowledge may, therefore, present problems to the researcher in that it involves 'artistry', which cannot easily be put into words. Observational methods are preferable, but failing this, in-depth unstructured interviews may suffice, providing that it is recognized that they do not provide a totally unproblematic version of reality. However, practitioner knowledge also constitutes an untapped resource for cooperative enquiry (Eraut 1985). Joint ventures could include: collaborative research projects, problem-oriented seminars and jointly planned programmes of continuing education.

Although Eraut is writing about teaching, these ideas fit with the so-called 'new paradigm' of research (Reason and Rowan, 1981; Lincoln and Guba,1985). Heron (1981), examining the philosophical basis for the new paradigm, remarks that the researcher cannot assume themselves to be intelligent and self directing, then apply different assumptions to the research subjects; in the new paradigm, subjects become partners in the research and are thereby protected from exploitation and alienation. Heron also suggests that the researcher should consider the value system of the researched, since otherwise only 'alienated pseudo-truths' will be produced. New paradigm research thus resembles the interactionist tradition, in which the meaning of the situation is crucial, although Carr and Kemmis (1986) argue that it is also important to recognize the limits imposed upon us in our practice setting. As Schon (1987) suggested, the new-paradigm approaches descend to the swamp of important problems, to which the rigours of the traditional positivist model do not apply. A similar perspective is taken by feminist researchers (Oakley, 1981; Graham, 1984), who argue that traditional approaches to research embody power differentials between researcher and researched. The approach advocated by Eraut is not only in tune with new-paradigm research, but also with recent developments in human resource management, such as quality assurance and job enrichment (Caves, 1988; Sisson, 1989). Such approaches are generally based on Maslow's (1943) concept of self-actualizing man which, despite its critics (Butler, 1986) has proved enduringly popular both in management and in clinical practice. There is, however, a contrary trend in quality assurance, in which detailed measurement is required. Fish (1991) argues strongly against this trend which, she says, results in a simplistic 'sum of the parts'; not everything can be measured.

IMPLICATIONS FOR PRACTICE

The work of Benner and Schon has proved to be hugely popular in nursing, undoubtedly partly because of the 'feel good factor' we get from seeing practitioners valued. We do, however, need to consider the extent to which we are currently able to put into practice the rigorous demands of the practicum as outlined by Schon, and it is not certain that we have really looked seriously at how (or whether) the situations described by Schon translate into our own work settings. There are also threats as well as opportunities in the current situation. In health care practice we have tended to devalue particularistic craft-based knowledge in favour of the more generalizable discipline-based knowledge, and it is important not to over-accentuate this trend. Hirst (1979) sounded a warning note here when he commented that we do not rehearse what we have learned from academic disciplines before acting. These disciplines refine our common sense and the knowledge base of professional practice should be acquired by working alongside practitioners, then analysing that experience with the help of the disciplines. There is, however, a tension between those who advocate the 'tough-minded' option of 'hard subject matter' and those who support the 'tender-minded' art of practice; teaching practice as a science would, it is argued, enable practitioners to become more confident about their practice in a world and health service dominated by the high value placed on science.

These proposals illustrate the fragility of the approaches to professional knowledge discussed in this chapter. It is also important to safeguard the means by which theory and practice can be integrated, such as lecturer practitioner posts. In the NHS, there has been a discrepancy between espoused theory and theory in use on a grand scale; the clinical grading review in nursing, for example, which was initially set up to recognize the value of clinical experience and provide a proper clinical career structure, appears to have had the opposite effect (Dyson, 1992). Lastly, we may be undergoing what Schon has termed 'the squeeze play', in which the resurgence of technical rationality, the constriction on professional autonomy and the emphasis on value for money in both education and health care combine to squeeze out the very idea of education for professional wisdom or artistry, or their application in practice. The current debate over skills mix illustrates how difficult it is for practitioners to defend their practice if it is defined only in terms of tasks and the importance of proposing other ways of looking at practice. These issues need to be addressed urgently if Benner and Schon's work is to be anything other than a brief fashion in curriculum documents, and this will require practitioner researchers and writers to examine and promote their practitioner knowledge as a legitimate way of informing practice.

REFERENCES

Agor, W. (1989) *Intuition in Organisations: Leading and Managing Productively*, Sage, Menlo Park CA.

Argyris, C. and Schon, D. (1974) *Theory in Practice*, Jossey-Bass, San Francisco.

Ash, E. (1992) The personal–professional interface in learning: towards reflective education. *Journal of Interprofessional Care*, 6(3), 261–71.

Atkinson, P., Reid, M. and Sheldrake, P. (1977) Medical mystique. *Sociology of Work and Occupations*, 4(3), 243–80.

Becker, H. and Geer, B. (1957) Participant observation and interviewing; a comparison. *Human Organisation*, 16, 28–32.

Benner, P. (1984) *From Novice to Expert*, Addison Wesley, Menlo Park CA.

Berger, P. and Luckmann, T. (1967) *The Social Construction of Reality*, Penguin, Harmondsworth.

Berman, M. (1990) *Coming to Our Senses*, Bantam New Age Books, New York.

Bhaskar, R. and Simon, H. (1977) Problem solving in semantically rich domains: an example of engineering thermodynamics. *Cognitive Science*, 1, 193–215.

Boud, D. (1989) Introduction, in *Making Sense of Experiential Learning: Diversity in Theory and Practice*, (eds T. Warner Weil and I. McGill), SRHE/Open University Press, Milton Keynes.

Broudy, H., Smith, B. and Burnett, J. (1964) *Democracy and Excellence in American Secondary Education*, Rand McNally, Chicago,

Butler, G. (1986) *Organisation and Management*, Prentice Hall, New York.

Carper, B. (1978) Fundamental patterns of knowing in nursing. *Advances in Nursing Science*, 1(1), 13–23.

Carr, W. and Kemmis, S. (1986) *Becoming Critical*, Falmer, Lewes.

Caves, R. (1988) Consultative methods for extracting expert knowledge about professional competence, in *Professional Competence and Quality Assurance in the Caring Professions*, (ed R. Ellis), Chapman and Hall, London.

Chenitz, W. and Swanson, J. (1986) *From Practice to Grounded Theory: Qualitative Research in Nursing*, Addison Wesley, Wokingham.

Close, F. (1991) *Too Hot to Handle: The Story of the Race for Cold Fusion*, W.H. Allen, London.

Collins, H. (1974) The TEA set; tacit knowledge and scientific networks. *Science Studies*, 4, 165–85.

Dingwall, R. (1977) *The Social Organisation of Health Visitor Training*, Croom Helm, London.

Dreistadt, R. (1968) An analysis of the use of analogies and metaphors in science. *Journal of Psychology*, 68, 97–116.

Dreyfus, H. and Dreyfus, S. (1986) *Mind Over Machine*, Free Press, New York.

Dreyfus, S. (1981) Formal models versus human situational understanding: inherent limitations on the modelling of business expertise. *Office Technology and People*, 1, 133–55.

Dyson, J. (1992) The importance of practice. *Nursing Times*, **88**, 44–6.
Elias, N. (1978) *The Civilising Process*, Basil Blackwell, Oxford.
Emerson, J. (1963) *The Social Function of Humor in a Hospital Setting*, Unpublished PhD thesis, University of California, Berkeley.
Eraut, M. (1982) What is learned in in-service education and how? A knowledge use perspective. *British Journal of In-Service Education*, **9**(1), 6–13.
Eraut, M. (1985) Knowledge creation and knowledge use in professional contexts. *Studies in Higher Education*, **10**(2), 117–33.
Fielding, P. (1986) *Attitudes Revisited*, RCN, London.
Fielding, N. and Lee, R. (1991) *Using Computers in Qualitative Research*, Sage, London.
Fish, D. (1991) But can you prove it? Quality assurance and the reflective practitioner. *Assessment and Evaluation in Higher Education*, **16**(1), 22–36.
Freidson, E. (1971) *Profession of Medicine*, Dodd Mead, New York.
Freidson, E. (1986) *Professional Powers: a Study of the Institutionalization of Formal Knowledge*, University of Chicago Press, Chicago.
Graham, H. (1984) Surveying through stories, in *Social Researching: Politics, Problems and Practice*, (eds C.Bell and H. Roberts), Routledge and Kegan Paul, London, pp. 70–87.
Harding, S. (1991) *Whose Science? Whose Knowledge? Thinking from Women's Lives*, Cornell University Press, New York.
Heron, J. (1981) Philosophical basis for the new paradigm, in *Human Enquiry: A Sourcebook of New Paradigm Research*, (eds P. Reason and J. Rowan), John Wiley, New York, pp. 19–35.
Hirst, P. (1979) Professional studies in initial teacher education: some conceptual issues, in *Professional Studies for Teaching*, (eds R. Alexander and E. Wormald), SRHE, Guildford, pp. 15–29.
Isenberg, D. (1991) How senior managers think, in *Creative Management*, (ed J. Henry), Sage, London.
Jamous, H. and Peloille, B. (1970) The French university–hospital system, in *Professions and Professionalization*, (ed J. Jackson), Cambridge University Press, Cambridge, pp. 111–52.
Jones, J. (1989) The verbal protocol: a research technique for nursing. *Journal of Advanced Nursing*, **14**, 1062–70.
Kaufmann, G. (1980) *Imagery, Language and Cognition*, Norwegian University Press, Oslo.
Koestler, A. (1989) *The Act of Creation*, Arkana, London.
Kolb, D. (1984) *Experiential Learning*, Prentice Hall, Englewood Cliffs.
Kratz, C. (1978) *Care of the Long Term Sick in the Community*, Churchill Livingstone, Edinburgh.
Lawler, J. (1991) *Behind the Screens*, Churchill Livingstone, Edinburgh.
Lincoln, Y. and Guba, E. (1985) *Naturalistic Enquiry*, Sage, Beverley Hills.
Macleod, M. (1990) *Experience in Everyday Nursing Practice: a Study of 'Experienced' Ward Sisters*, Unpublished PhD thesis, University of Edinburgh.
Maslow, A. (1943) A theory of motivation. *Psychological Review*, **50**(4), 370–96.
Miles, M. (1979) Qualitative data as an attractive nuisance. *Administrative Science Quarterly*, **24**, 590–601.
Mintzberg, H. (1991) Planning on the left side and managing on the right, in *Creative Management*, (ed J. Henry), Sage, London, pp. 58–71.
Oakeshott, M. (1962) *Rationalism in Politics, and Other Essays*, Methuen, London.
Oakley, A.(1981) Interviewing women: a contradiction in terms, in *Doing Feminist Research*, (ed H. Roberts), Routledge and Kegan Paul, London.
Ornstein, R. (1975) *The Psychology of Consciousness*, W.H. Freeman, San Francisco.

Polanyi, M. (1958) *Personal Knowledge: Towards a Post Critical Philosophy*, Routledge and Kegan Paul, London.

Polanyi, M. (1967) *The Tacit Dimension*, Routledge and Kegan Paul, London.

Reason, P. and Rowan, J. (1981) *Human Enquiry*, John Wiley, New York.

Reed, J. (1994) Phenomenology without phenomena: a discussion of the use of phenomenology to examine expertise in long term care of elderly patients. *Journal of Advanced Nursing*, **19**, 336–341.

Rew, L. and Barrow, E. (1987) Intuition: a neglected hallmark of nursing knowledge. *Advances in Nursing Science*, **10**, 49–62.

Schon, D. (1987) *Educating the Reflective Practitioner*, Jossey Bass, San Francisco.

Simon, H. (1969) *Administrative Behaviour*, 2nd edn, Macmillan, New York.

Sisson, K. (1989) *Personnel Management in Britain*, Basil Blackwell, Oxford.

Smith, P. (1992) *The Emotional Labour of Nursing: How Nurses Care*, Macmillan, London.

Turner, B. (1992) *Regulating Bodies: Essays in Medical Sociology*, Routledge, London.

Vaughan, B. (1992) The nature of nursing knowledge, in *Knowledge for Nursing Practice*, (eds K. Robinson and B. Vaughan), Butterworth-Heinemann, London.

White, E. (1952) *Charlotte's Web*, Harper and Row, New York.

Younger, J. (1990) Literary works as a mode of knowing. *Image: Journal of Nursing Scholarship*, **22**(1), 39–43.

CHAPTER 3

ractitioner knowledge in practitioner research

Jan Reed

INTRODUCTION

One of the biggest issues facing practitioner researchers is the way in which their practitioner knowledge and identity affects the collection of data. Although it may be possible, when planning research, to maintain a degree of distance from the self, when actually in the field the self and its values, knowledge and habits have a disturbing tendency to intrude on the research. Many practitioner researchers become anxious about this bias and struggle to overcome, suppress or control it. The anxiety partly arises because the self and, in particular, the practitioner knowledge that it manifests, is seen as subjective and therefore out of place in an endeavour which is traditionally valued for its objective scientific status.

Maturana (1991), however, has remarked that 'Science is a human activity and must be understood as such because it is in the domain of human relations that it exists' (Maturana, 1991, p. 30). This deceptively simple comment sums up the main theme of this chapter and one of the main theses of this book: that research is done by people and to understand it it is necessary to understand the people who create or construct it. If the research is done by practitioners rather than traditional academic researchers, then part of this understanding will come from a discussion of the practitioner knowledge (in a wide sense, including experiential knowledge and values) that the researcher has, which will be different from that displayed by the non-practitioner.

In non-practitioner research this notion of research as being socially constructed by individuals is being increasingly articulated. The idea that there is some truth which exists independently of those who perceive it was quite thoroughly demolished by Kant, in his *Critique of Pure Reason*, in which he argued that if there is a reality out there we can never know it in itself – we can only know it as we perceive it. Extending this argument to the philosophy of science, the notion that it is possible or even desirable to attempt to disentangle facts from the persons who perceive them, becomes nonsensical.

Murphy and Longino (1992) have graphically described this idea of objective science, which they see as being based on a dualistic distinction between fact and value: 'Whereas the human element is replete with prejudices, quantitative methods are believed to be free from these impediments. By adhering to algorithmic or step wise instructions that do not require interpretation, direct access is gained to facts'. They go on to describe the way in which such value-free science proceeds:

> . . . the image is created that volition has no role to play in research, because a study is portrayed to consist simply of various technical operations. Those who are involved in gathering data, therefore, are often lulled into thinking that they are detached observers of social life.

This ideal of valid research as being a simple matter of technical operations, in which values or interpretation play no part, has been challenged even in those sciences usually thought of as the pinnacles of objectivity, namely physics, chemistry and mathematics. Knorr-Cetina (1983), for example, has described how scientific conclusions emerge not simply from a technical analysis of research results, but from interaction and debate between scientists. Thom (1990) has argued that even in mathematics, surely the most value-free of all sciences, mathematical operations are context-bound – in other words that concepts such as probability are only meaningful in context.

If we move from pre-Kantian notions of a reality out there that is independent of our own experience of it, then we are forced to pay attention to our involvement in the development or construction of knowledge. To this end, Steier (1991b) has suggested thinking of research as a reflexive process, involving 'second-order cybernetics'. First-order cybernetics can be thought of as the observation of social processes, whereas second-order cybernetics incorporates the observer and becomes the study of the study of social processes. By explicitly paying attention to the observer, Steier argues that the observer takes some responsibility for the process – research data and conclusions can no longer be attributed to impersonal technical procedures.

Steier also has an interesting point to make about the term reflexive. It can, he says, be used in two ways: first to suggest immediate reflex responses, and secondly to suggest a contemplative response, what he calls small-circuit and long-circuit reflexivity. Both types of reflexivity are important in practitioner research: immediate responses are partly a product of practitioner knowledge and help the practitioner researcher to immerse themselves in situations. Many of the ways in which practitioner researchers respond to research settings are of this order.

Contemplative responses, however, are also important to allow 'an active questioning of the assumptions which make a small-circuit reflexivity in action possible' (Steier, 1991b, p. 164). Without labouring the electrical metaphor too much, many of the debates discussed in this chapter can be seen as being about the relationship between small- and long-circuit reflexivity.

To illustrate these points about how knowledge can be seen as socially constructed and how reflexivity has a place in practitioner research, we can use an illustration from one of the author's own studies, when conducting observation for the first time (Reed, 1989). At the first observation session, the researcher turned up on a ward for the elderly at 7.30 in the morning, equipped with blank sheets of paper and several pens, anxious that she would not be able to write quickly enough to record all the events which would occur and which were relevant to the area of study (the nursing assessment of the mobility status of elderly patients). After 2 hours of standing around the ward feeling uncomfortable and useless, the sheets of paper were as blank as they had been at the beginning of the session. What had been anticipated as a dress rehearsal for the observation had turned out to be a flop.

Discussing this with an academic supervisor, who had no experience of nursing, the researcher stated that nothing interesting had happened. When asked to describe what had happened, in layman's terms, the supervisor was immediately interested. In the space of 2 hours, the nurses had got 24 patients out of bed, toileted, washed and dressed them and given them their medicines and breakfasts. When asked for details about what, for example, toileting involved, the researcher found it difficult to describe, but as the description unfolded many questions were raised, mainly along the lines of 'Why do they do it that way?' These were questions which had not occurred to the researcher, because so much about the nurses' activities had been taken for granted. To an outsider, however, they seemed mysterious and fascinating and worthy of inquiry.

This outsider construction, therefore, was a useful counterbalance to the researcher's tendency to see the activities of the nurses as not very interesting. As the researcher had been involved in the same activities the day before the observation session, and indeed carried them out the next day, what had happened had been simply routine – this is what you would expect nurses to do at this time of the day. When pushed into asking questions about why these things were happening, the potential of routine work as a source of data became more apparent.

The fruitless observation session was also discussed with nursing colleagues, who were interested to know how it had gone. The reaction to the statement 'nothing much happened' was again met with questions, but of a different nature from those of the supervisor. Colleagues' questions were along the lines of What on earth were they doing then –

the morning is one of the busiest times on the ward? One more telling response came from a nurse who said, 'Well what do you expect on there – they're a lazy lot.'

Juxtaposing these two constructions – the insider and the outsider – it became clear that something had happened on that day, but that how it was described or thought about differed depending on the audience. The nurses had carried out complex and demanding care which to the outsider looked puzzling because it had no apparent rationale, but to the insider was an accepted and legitimate way to work – the suggestion that the nurses had done nothing was puzzling because it suggested a very peculiar way of working, which conflicted with their expectations of practice and also their notions of good practice. Putting these two responses together, the decision was made to record these routine behaviours and to explore the meaning they had for the nurses.

In practitioner research these insider and outsider constructions cannot always be conveniently lodged or accorded to particular persons – it is more often the case that as practitioner researchers we move between these perspectives in our own thinking. Sometimes we see things in a new light as researchers, decontextualized and strange, and sometimes we understand things as practitioners, contextualized and familiar. It is tempting, however, to suppress or fail to use one of the positions open to us, and because of the lack of guidance in methodology texts it is likely to be the practitioner view which is lost, or regarded as a threat to the purity of the research. This seems to be a tragic waste of knowledge, and so this chapter hopes to explore this practitioner knowledge and the role that it can play in research more fully, so that it can be used rather than discarded.

The chapter is loosely organised according to the chronological sequence of research stages. It deals first with practitioner knowledge in selecting research settings, then in developing research relationships, and then in data collection and analysis. As in research, however, the boundaries between these stages are by no means clear, and there is a certain amount of overlap between sections, but in the interests of intelligibility we have tried to keep to this structure. The most important part of research, developing aims and questions, is discussed in Chapter 1; the nature of practitioner knowledge was covered in Chapter 2. Ideally, this chapter should be read after the first two, but readers should find enough discussion to make our ideas intelligible.

USING PRACTITIONER KNOWLEDGE IN SELECTING RESEARCH SETTINGS

The success of any research project depends in part on the ability of the researcher to select and identify relevant and appropriate samples and fields from which to collect data. This selection process is usually based on identifying variables which are important to the study, and matching up samples to these variables. Practitioner knowledge is important in both these decisions: what is important and where these things are to be found.

Take, for example, a study which is attempting to look at the ways in which practitioners deal with dying patients, perhaps in the way that they break bad news. One thing which is immediately apparent is that breaking bad news is not necessarily a decision that individual practitioners make, and that there are often policies or unwritten rules about how this is done and by whom. In addition, there are also differences in the way that practitioners work which will affect the degree to which they are able to break bad news, or even the likelihood that they will be aware that there is bad news to be broken.

Randomly sampling staff in a health authority and asking them questions, therefore, is, as the practitioner knows, likely to produce meaningless results. Those practitioners in situations where they have only intermittent contact with patients, for example dietitians, may feel with some justification that they are not the appropriate people to break bad news, and they will demonstrate a corresponding reluctance to do it. Other staff may work in settings where the diagnosis of a terminal condition is not disclosed to patients because of medical disapproval, and to make this disclosure will provoke censure, if not disciplinary action. Again, their responses will indicate reluctance to break bad news, not because they do not think it right but because they are not 'allowed' to.

These different attitudes to disclosure, and their origins, can be explored through the use of sensitive research methods and data analysis, but again this is dependent on the researcher being aware that such sensitivity is needed. For the outsider, who is not aware of different ways of practice or the subtle differences in the way that death is dealt with in health care organizations, there may not be such awareness. For the insider, such knowledge can inform the study from the start, shaping the research question and the sample selection. An insider might decide that because of the differences in practice it is more appropriate to ask questions about the way in which these differences affect breaking bad news, and choose the sample or setting accordingly.

The lack of insider knowledge in sampling is a serious problem for studies if they are to produce results that are meaningful to practitioners (this may, of course, not be the aim – see Chapter 1). We can all think of studies we have read which seem to us to be naive and misguided because this knowledge has not been used. A study which looks at discharge planning, for example, and fails to distinguish between long-stay, terminal care and acute care settings misses important points about the purpose of different types of care. A study on patients' feelings about privacy which does not take into account the design of clinical areas (for example 'Nightingale' wards, mixed wards, single cubicle wards) again seems naive. This naiveté, although often prized by researchers as leading to challenging research, is also likely to produce research which does not take into account the complexities of the practice world, often because these complexities are not known.

Practitioner knowledge, then, can make important contributions to the planning and design of studies. This is not only a general knowledge of the way things are, but it can also be a specific and detailed knowledge of particular settings. Looking at the process of rehabilitation, for example, and the way in which a multidisciplinary team works, an insider can select settings that cover a range of different approaches, from the autocratic consultant who assumes team leadership but pays only lip-service to the principles of team working, to the democratic unit where team leadership rotates among different professions. This selection depends on insider knowledge, often gained in ways which are viewed as unorthodox by methodology texts, for example by working in clinical areas, from chatting to colleagues in the canteen, from listening to people who have been patients in different settings. This is not quite the same process that occurs when researchers use participant observation, because it is not always knowledge gained for research purposes, but is knowledge gained by virtue of the fact that the practitioner is part of the organization as a worker there.

Using practitioner knowledge in research design fits in many ways with Glaser and Strauss's (1967) notion of theoretical sampling, in which samples are chosen not because of the concern with generalization but because they afford an opportunity to develop theory (Glaser and Strauss, 1967). What is often forgotten, however, in discussions of theoretical sampling, is that in order to do this the researcher must not only have a clear idea of how they wish to develop theory, but also of the people or settings likely to help them to do this. In the study by Reed (1989) mentioned above, where data collection had initially begun in long-term care of the elderly wards, the data indicated that the function of these wards – to house those who were unlikely to be discharged – had an effect on the way that nurses saw assessment. To develop this theory it was necessary to look at another care of the elderly ward which had a different function, in order to see whether attitudes towards assessment differed within this specialty or were the same in different types of ward. Because the researcher knew the system it was easy to identify a suitable ward for the study; without this knowledge, the official descriptions of the wards would not have been much help.

Developing this type of insider knowledge, however, is not simply a matter of spending time in practice – we are not arguing that there is an 'osmotic process' of knowledge acquisition taking place. Practitioners cannot develop knowledge simply by being in practice for a long time – as if knowledge could be passively absorbed by simple physical contact with the practice environment. We can all probably think of colleagues (or even, in some circumstances, ourselves) who have spent time in practice but do not seem to have learned much from it.

There is, of course, the argument that we may well have absorbed knowledge without knowing that we have done so. Knowledge that we are not aware we have, however, is of limited use in explicating the processes of practitioner research – it needs to be brought out and made public, so that its strengths and limitations can be explored.

This suggests that practitioner knowledge should be actively and consciously explored, examined and developed for it to form a viable basis for practitioner research. This active process, which we have called 'attentive practice', is exemplified in many chapters in this book (see, for example, Chapters 8 and 9), where practitioners have paid attention to what is happening in practice. This is more than simply noticing puzzling, unexpected or striking events, but involves further active contemplation and exploration, activities which, in the examples in this book, have led to the development of systematic studies.

ROLES AND RELATIONSHIPS IN PRACTITIONER RESEARCH

When choosing research settings, we have argued that practitioner researchers can use knowledge they have because they are practitioners, either general knowledge about practice or specific knowledge about settings. This practitioner knowledge is also apparent when entering into a research setting, not simply in the way that it informs the social niceties of becoming accepted, but also because it is likely to be the aspect of the researcher that is most easily identified by research participants. Whereas the research knowledge that the practitioner researcher has may not be understood by participants, the knowledge that they are thought to have as practitioners can become a focal point for developing research relationships.

Pearsall (1965) has suggested that:

> the pull towards complete participation in the already familiar capacity of [practitioner] is likely to be strong, the more so because others find the . . . role clearer than that of scientific observer.

This is a particular problem for those who are, in effect, researching their own practice in their usual setting – it becomes difficult to decide whether one is there as a researcher or as a practitioner, and the tensions between the two ('between disinterested observation and interested action'; Pearsall, 1965) can seem almost insurmountable. Even those who are researching the practice of colleagues away from their practice setting can feel these tensions, largely because their previous experience of clinical settings has been as a practitioner and this acclimatization cannot be readily abandoned simply because one is collecting data.

The other side of the coin is, of course, the expectations of research participants. The presence of a researcher is not a normal part of everyday practice and people will spend some time in placing the intruder, by asking questions and 'checking them out'. The researcher is more likely to become a practitioner who is doing research, rather than a researcher who is a practitioner, simply because the practitioner role is better understood and more familiar to participants and so they will find practitioner-oriented questions easier to ask. These may range from questions about training and experience to questions about current practice. The authors have both been asked about the methods we use in dressing patients' wounds, or for advice on patient care. Sometimes the practitioner role can become so prominent that the researcher is expected to act as one of the workforce – this is fine if you are trying to be a close participant, but difficult to manage if you are not. Refusing to behave as a practitioner can be interpreted as hostile, and not joining in practice can be seen as suspicious. If the participants' prior experience of research has been a negative one – for example some form of quality assurance which has produced critical results – then participants may see any reluctance to join them as being evidence that you are against them.

These observations suggest that whatever role the researcher has decided upon, this cannot be enforced on participants – some negotiation will occur. Both researcher and participant may well have in mind some ideal role, but the reality is likely to be less clear cut. Researchers may wish to adopt a role which allows them access to data as the research demands, but which does not encumber them with obligations that distract from the research. Participants may wish a researcher to be positive about their practice and preferably not get in the way of their work. It is unlikely that these different demands can be resolved absolutely, or indeed that any research role will be fixed at all. As Pearsall has pointed out:

> People tend to handle the vaguely . . . disturbing presence of a difficult-to-place stranger by alternately pulling him into their ranks where he would be subject to group sanctions, and pushing him out again when his behaviour becomes too unpredictable or suspicious.

These vacillations may occur in the role of any researcher, whether practitioner or not, but they are potentiated by the existence of a

practitioner identity. The practitioner role is so well known to participants that it forms the basis of any ideas they may have of the
researcher.

Attempts to drop the practitioner role – perhaps to deny or disguise it
– are tempting. One argument made for doing this is that researchers
want to be treated like an ordinary person, in other words that they are
uncomfortable with their practitioner identity and feel that it may bias
responses to them. This argument, of course, recognizes that people's
responses are affected by the person they are responding to, but it does
raise the question of why being responded to as an ordinary person is
better than being responded to as a practitioner.

Attempts to disguise practitioner experience are often unsuccessful
and even unethical. Practitioner knowledge is often so hidden, even
from the person who has it, that they cannot control their displays of
knowledge – they use terminology or ask questions which betray their
understanding. Apart from this problem of being 'found out', there is
also an ethical problem in such deception – to be less than honest about
so important a part of one's research seems to be an unwarranted
deception. If the research depends, as most does, on the informed
consent of participants, then surely withholding such details gives less
than adequate information on which to base this consent. Furthermore,
if the research is being conducted in order to develop practice, then such
an exercise of power does not fit with ideas of equipping practitioners
with the knowledge to change things – it simply relegates them to being
passive recipients of knowledge.

Roles and relationships in practitioner research appear to be confusing
and problematic. They are probably no more so than roles in other types
of research, but the problems are rather differently cast. Whereas the
problem for the traditional researcher is in gaining familiarity with the
field (whether they are qualitative researchers or quantitative, they still
need some knowledge about the setting that they are studying), the
practitioner researcher may well feel that the problem is too much
familiarity. This familiarity may confuse the research, not only because it
intrudes upon the research role that they desire to adopt, but also
because it can prevent them from seeing practice with fresh eyes. Their
data collection and analysis therefore runs the risk of doing little but
perpetuate existing views of practice.

Because of this, practitioner researchers must make explicit their
position and the attendant concerns, interests and views that they have,
so that they can be debated by not only research participants and
readers, but also by the researchers themselves. Many of the contributors in this book (see Chapters 5, 6, 7 and 8, for example) attempt to
make explicit their practitioner perspective in their accounts of their
research. This openness, as they acknowledge, led to a clearer understanding and a challenging of their positions, leading to much more

critical analysis than would have been possible if they had not been acknowledged.

PRACTITIONER KNOWLEDGE IN DATA COLLECTION AND ANALYSIS

As the discussion above indicates, practitioner knowledge forms an important foundation for the planning of research and the management of research roles, even before data collection has begun. The impact of practitioner knowledge is also apparent during data collection and analysis. This is the case not only when the practitioner researcher is engaged in formal research strategies, such as interviews or question-naires, but also when they are engaged in their everyday practice. Every day practitioners collect information, develop understanding and create theories which are directed to their practice and derive from it. If they are concurrently carrying out research, then the insights gained through practice will have an impact on the research too. It is sometimes difficult to record this process: whereas conventional research reporting tra-ditions give a framework for describing formal research methods and their results, the informal data collection which sits alongside this pro-cess is much more difficult to incorporate into the research account.

Jean Davies (Chapter 8) describes this informal data collection by using the term 'practitioner observation', which she likens to the better-known idea of participant observation described in many research text-books. Like participant observation, practitioner observation involves the collection of many different types of data, which present themselves to the researcher in the course of their interaction with research partici-pants. The difference between the two lies in the position of the researcher – if the role is a simple research one, then data can be tailored to the research aims, but in practitioner observation data are collected primarily for practice purposes. This can result in the practitioner researcher being flooded with data which are not immediately relevant to the research, but it also means that data can be collected which provide a broader basis for the research, or which can act as a counter-balance to a narrow definition of the research aims.

As we have described it, practitioner observation can take place as an integral part of the research or as a background to it, but it will always take place. It seems, therefore, that practitioner researchers would be well advised to acknowledge its place in the generation of research and to incorporate data obtained in this way in their research accounts.

Whatever the methods chosen in practitioner research, the business of asking questions, recording and analysing data is affected by the prior experience of the researcher. In interviews, for example, practitioner researchers will ask questions which derive from their understanding of practice and of what is important to it. In an interview about admission policies, for example, a practitioner researcher might ask questions about the different ways in which emergency and waiting list admissions are handled, about consultant preferences and how the timing of the admission and the differences in ward activities and staffing affect patient reception.

An observational study will be governed by practitioner knowledge too, but this will determine not only what is observed, but how it is recorded and analysed. Practitioners tend to see the behaviour of others in global terms – rather than a microanalysis of activity, behaviours can be put together into bigger units which make sense to the practitioner. Rather than recording an event as 'X approaches patient carrying tray. Says "hello, lunch time". Sits down beside patient and proceeds to cut up food. Takes a spoonful of food and holds it in front of patient's mouth. Patient opens mouth. X puts food into it', a practitioner researcher is more likely to simply record that 'X feeds patient', because this is what that sequence of behaviours means to the practitioner researcher.

There are problems and advantages to this analytic leap. By grouping activities into professionally meaningful units, a process which can happen almost automatically, the practitioner researcher can certainly record data more quickly and, depending on the purpose of the research, more usefully. The problem lies, however, in the lack of attention paid to detail, which may well generate new insights. In the example above, the finely detailed record of the event observed allows some interesting points to emerge. The lack of conversation, for example, seems rather strange, as does the passive behaviour of the patient – how are mealtimes regarded by the participants?

The analytic leaps made by practitioner researchers, therefore, can simply perpetuate their existing views of practice, rather than challenging them. Another example could be found among the many studies of patient–staff communication in which observation checklists are frequently constructed around the notion of types of interaction. Typically these types are given titles such as 'therapeutic', 'instrumental' and 'social'. The researcher then proceeds to treat these titles as unproblematic, indeed self-evident, and classifies communication events accordingly. Usually communication will be found to be mainly instrumental and social, with very little of it being therapeutic.

This seems to be an uncritical misuse of practitioner knowledge. Although the characteristics of each criterion may be explained in the study, their justification is often weak and depends upon the notion that communication can be categorized in this way, that every interaction falls into one category. The titles of the categories themselves and the preceding discussions are value-laden, in that it is assumed that therapeutic interaction is more valuable and important than any other form.

Finally, it is assumed that these types of communication can be easily recognized by anyone and practitioner knowledge is not acknowledged – these checklists do not depend on professional experience and are therefore pure and scientific.

If we start to acknowledge and explore practitioner knowledge, however, this model of communication is challenged. We can start to think about interactions that we have had with patients which do not fit this schema. We may, for example, remember instances where our interaction may well have looked social but had therapeutic intent – MacLeod gives an example of this when she described a ward sister discussing fashion with a young woman who had just had a colostomy (MacLeod, 1990). This could be classified as social communication but was therapeutic in intent, as it indicated to the patient that she could maintain an interest in fashion, like other women of her age, despite her colostomy.

We may also think about long-term interaction strategies that we have used with patients, which snapshot research methods would not necessarily identify. Hunt (1991) gives an account of such approaches when she discusses the strategies that nurses caring for terminally ill patients in the community use to develop closeness. Their initial interactions with patient and family are not ostensibly therapeutic, but are directed towards building up a friendly, informal relationship which will allow the discussion of death and bereavement to take place later on in the relationship. A simplistic model may classify initial conversations as only social, but they are inherently therapeutic.

MacLeod's and Hunt's work illustrates a reflective use of practitioner knowledge. Instead of jumping to conclusions, they were sufficiently aware of practice to recognize the need for critical research, which would illuminate the fine detail of practice. Perhaps most importantly, part of their research aim was to further the understanding of practitioner–client relationships, in a way which would be useful to the development of practice. This governed not only the way in which they collected data, but also the way they analysed it, searching for examples of skilled practice.

Data analysis in practitioner research is affected by practitioner knowledge in much the same way as data collection is. In fact, it is important not to separate data collection and analysis too much, as they are mutually dependent. The way in which data are recorded largely determines the way they can be analysed, and the way in which it is intended to analyse data shapes how they are collected. This is perhaps most clearly seen in quantitative research, in which the form and type of data collected specifies the type of analysis that can be conducted, but the principle remains true in qualitative work.

Data analysis, therefore, is closely linked to the aims of the research and the methods used, and if these are determined by practitioner knowledge then so will analytic processes be. Prior practitioner experience is an important part of deciding what is important in the data and also what it means. Consider, for example, the following data collected in one study (Reed, 1989):

> *Interviewer*: How would you describe the work that goes on in this ward?
> *Respondent*: Oh, I think it's wonderful, the staff really work hard, they do a wonderful job.

At first glance this seems like an unequivocally supportive statement, but in the context in which it occurred it was perhaps more ambivalent. The respondent was a consultant and the ward was a long-term care of the elderly ward which attracted few visits from medical staff. Understanding the multidisciplinary aspects of care and the significance that medical interest can have for the morale of other staff, and the usual lack of popularity that long-term care of the elderly has for medical staff, these comments can be seen as either dismissive or patronizing. Thus in analysing these data these comments were not coded simply as positive views of medical staff, but were discussed in the light of their ambiguity.

This interpretation took place against a background of data which were analysed in the light of insider knowledge, but this type of knowledge needs to be carefully handled – it can, on occasion, become a substitute for analysis. Consider the following exchange from the same research:

> *Researcher*: How would you describe this ward?
> *Respondent*: Well, it's not really a geriatric ward, it's really more like a medical ward.
> *Researcher*: In what way?
> *Respondent*: Well, there's a lot going on, you know.
> *Researcher*: Right.

In this exchange, shared values and language between researcher and respondent led to several things being said without exciting comment, for example the phrases 'not really a geriatric ward' and 'like a medical ward' were a well understood way of describing and classifying clinical areas. When this interview was transcribed, however, these phrases became less than self-evident, and instead of being coded according to obvious meaning were explored further in subsequent interviews, to determine what they stood for. In fact, the result was quite surprising to the researcher, whose experience of medical wards had been quite tedious, and who enjoyed care of the elderly. What the nurses meant when they described a ward as being like a medical ward was that it was busy, interesting and cure-orientated, and that a geriatric ward was seen as boring.

There is a limit, however, to how far the practitioner researcher can go in questioning shared experience, especially, as we discussed above, as their practice experience is an important part of their relationship with participants. Concerned about this apparent uncritical acceptance of respondents statements, the researcher above tried to adopt a more questioning approach to interview conversations. This led to exchanges which puzzled respondents, and increased their wariness of the researcher:

> *Respondent*: Well, when we do a toilet round, we can be really busy.
> *Interviewer*: Right. So what is a toilet round?
> *Respondent*: What do you mean, what is a toilet round? I thought you were a nurse. Why are you asking that?

Challenging assumptions, therefore, can only go so far, and if a challenging approach is taken too far it can seem as if the researcher is setting traps for respondents. It seems that some things must be taken for granted, but perhaps the important issue for the practitioner researcher is that they know when this is happening. All researchers take things for granted – a researcher from outside does not, for example, ask people what they mean by 'ward' or 'patient' or 'doctor' – some things are recognized as being shared knowledge, and indeed it is this which makes any form of conversation possible.

Because the practitioner researcher shares more with participants, however, it becomes even more important that they are aware of this and in data collection and analysis become sensitized to the way in which they are seeing data. It seems more likely that this will happen if practitioner researchers are aware of practitioner knowledge and the part that it can play in research, than if they either do not recognize it or attempt to suppress it.

CONCLUSION

Practitioner research is largely shaped by the experience and knowledge that researchers have acquired through practice. It is knowledge which cannot be easily discarded – although attempts can be made to do so, the success of such attempts is debatable. Still, attempts are made and this leads us to wonder why. Perhaps it is because practitioner knowledge has been seen as elusive, not codifiable and incommunicable. This contrasts with notions of scientific knowledge as being clearly identifiable, logical and assessable. Perhaps practitioner knowledge is knowledge which, because it has not been derived through research, is not seen as making an acceptable contribution to research.

This undervaluing of practitioner knowledge is perhaps more a reflection of practitioners' ideas of research than a reflection of research itself. All researchers would recognize that every research study begins with a basic grasp of the topic to be studied, and indeed many texts exhort researchers to develop this knowledge further by reading the literature and previous studies. Some texts, it is true, suggest that researchers should approach topics with an open mind, but an open mind is not necessarily an empty one. In other words, the issue is not whether the researcher knows something about the topic to be studied but whether they know what they know and whether they are prepared to regard this knowledge as provisional rather than fixed.

What we would suggest is important, therefore, is that practitioner researchers acknowledge the extent and the limitations of their practitioner knowledge and, most importantly, challenge it. This involves a process of reflecting over experiences that have given rise to knowledge and considering other interpretations or conclusions that could have been developed. This approach recognizes the importance of the self in creating and constructing knowledge, and the circumstances that led knowledge to be constructed in this particular way. This takes us away from the notion of enquiry as being about the search for some incontrovertible truth, untainted by human action, and enables us to better describe the processes of construction that we engage in.

Instead of presenting absolute facts, therefore, research should perhaps be saying 'this is what I saw in these circumstances'. This contrasts sharply with notions of depersonalized research, in which the person doing the research becomes of no consequence to, or even a contaminant of, the research. These ideas have been challenged in many areas of research, but are of even more importance in practitioner research where, as this chapter has tried to show, the person is crucially important to the way in which enquiry is construed and undertaken.

Adherents of the depersonalized research approach have argued that such a relativist position, where all knowledge is seen as socially constructed, devalues research and makes its conduct meaningless. As Steier(1991a) says in his discussion of research and social construction: '. . . a question that is often posed is: Why do research (if you cannot say anything about what is out there, and all research is self-reflexive?)' Steier's response, which reflects what has been said here about the importance of the researcher in research is: 'Why do research for which you must deny responsibility for what **you** have found?' (Steier, 1991a, p.10).

REFERENCES

Glaser, B. G. and Strauss, A. L. (1967) *The Discovery of Grounded Theory: Strategies for Qualititative Research*, Aldine Press, Chicago.
Hunt, M. (1991) Being friendly and informal; reflected in nurses', terminally ill patients' and relatives' conversations at home. *Journal of Advanced Nursing*, **16**, 929–38.

Knorr-Cetina, K. (1983) The ethnographic study of scientific work: towards a constructionist interpretation of science, in *Science Observed: Perspectives on the Social Study of Science*, (eds K. Knorr-Cetina and M. Mulkay), Sage, London, pp. 115–40.

MacLeod, M. L. P. (1990) *Experience in Everyday Nursing Practice: a Study of "Experienced" Surgical Ward Sisters*, Unpublished PhD thesis, University of Edinburgh.

Maturana, H. R. (1991) Science and daily life: the ontology of scientific explanations, in *Research and Reflexivity*, (ed F. Steier), Sage, London, pp.30–52.

Murphy, J.W. and Longino, C.F. Jr (1992) What is the justification for a qualitative approach to ageing studies? *Ageing and Society*, **12**, 143–56.

Pearsall, M. (1965) Participant observation as role and method in behavioural research. *Nursing Research*, *14*(1), 37–42.

Reed, L. (1989) *All Dressed Up and Nowhere to Go: Nursing Assessment in Geriatric Wards*, Unpublished PhD thesis, Newcastle Polytechnic.

Steier, F. (1991a) Introduction: research as self-reflexivity, self-reflexivity as social process, in *Research and Reflexivity*, (ed F. Steier), Sage, London, pp. 1–11.

Steier, F. (1991b) Reflexivity and methodology: an ecological constructionism, in *Research and Reflexivity*, (ed F. Steier), Sage, London, pp. 163–85.

Thom, R. (1990) *Semio Physics*, Addison Wesley, Redwood City CA.

CHAPTER 4

The contribution of inductive and deductive theory to the development of practitioner knowledge

Sue Procter

INTRODUCTION

The first two chapters of this book set out what we believe are the distinguishing characteristics of practitioner research. Briefly, in Chapter 1 we indicated that practitioner research was distinguished by the need to meet a professional agenda, the aim of improving practice and the use of 'insider' knowledge.

In Chapter 2, Liz Meerabeau discusses tacit knowledge and links this to debates about the validity of insider knowledge and the development of practitioner knowledge. A key problem to emerge from the discussions in these chapters is the problem of interpreting the data from the perspective of the 'insider'. This theme is further discussed in Chapter 3, where Jan Reed draws on literature from the philosophy of science to highlight the complex debate surrounding data interpretation in research. She concludes that the notion of 'value-free' research is something of a misnomer. Values are implicit in every research paradigm; however, the influence of values in informing the research process is more openly discussed in some research paradigms, e.g. new-paradigm research and feminist research, than in others, e.g. correlational research.

This chapter sets out to discuss one possible strategy for dealing with the issue of professional values and the interpretation of data in practitioner research. It discusses my attempt to deal with these issues in my own research (Procter, 1989b) and describes a method which evolved during the course of the research. This method drew heavily on the philosophy underpinning action research (Winter, 1987), although throughout the research process no attempt was made to undertake an action research project. In other words, the research did not set out to transform practice, merely to document it. The ensuing discussion raises some interesting questions, particularly in relation to traditional notions of qualitative and quantitative research. For this reason I will begin with a debate of these issues, before moving on to more specific consideration of practitioner research, using nursung, my own discipline, as an illustration of my points.

THE QUALITATIVE/QUANTITATIVE DEBATE REVISITED

At a simplistic level the distinction between qualitative and quantitative research is frequently couched in terms of the use of numbers, or quantification. Quantitative research implies quantification; therefore, any research that uses numbers must, by definition, be quantitative. Qualitative research, on the other hand, is distinguished by the use of narrative or descriptive quotations from or about the research subjects.

As Silverman (1985) has argued, however, this is a very superficial distinction which appears to rule out the use of descriptive statistics as method of presenting qualitative data. If, as Silverman suggests, qualitative research is about description, counting can be a very useful method of succinctly portraying or describing a mass of dense narrative. More importantly, perhaps, it can provide a method of checking the analysis to indicate the generality of the finding, within the data set, both to the reader and to the researcher. This does not exclude reporting on unusual or rare occurrences within the data. Instead, it indicates how generalized or rare a particular finding is, so giving a more substantive indication of the frequency of the occurrence on which the subsequent analysis is based. Rare or unusual findings may indeed highlight important avenues for further investigation.

It is possible to argue that the distinction between qualitative and quantitative research in relation to the use of numbers rests not with the use of numbers *per se*, but with the use of numbers for purpose of prediction. The epistemological tradition from which quantitative research derives is fundamentally about prediction. Prediction is based on notions of causal analysis. If we can identify the cause(s) of a given event we can predict the circumstances under which that event is likely to arise in the future.

In order to pursue this path quantitative research adopts a deductive stance towards the data. This means that key variables are distilled from previous research and developed into a hypothesis for testing. Although the hypothesis may be written in relation to variables, it is the theories that gave rise to the variables that the researchers are actually attempting to test (de Vaus, 1986). The strengths of this approach for the academic community are:

- It is intrinsically cumulative, as it builds on the results of previous research.
- It requires specialist knowledge of the area being researched.
- It facilitates the development of a research career based around the development of knowledge in a specialist field.

Consequently, quantitative researchers will frequently develop questionnaires or set up experiments which are designed to test out an underlying hypothesis. While making perfect sense to the researcher, they are often incomprehensible or meaningless to the research subject, who may feel that none of the responses from which they have to choose reflects their position or ideas. Alternatively, the research subject may feel that they want to qualify their response or elaborate on it and they may feel misrepresented if this desire is not met. From the researcher's point of view such data, although potentially interesting, are irrelevant in relation to the hypothesis they are currently testing.

It is at this point that qualitative researchers take issue with quantitative approaches to research, arguing that the denial of the research subject's position renders the research meaningless. It is only by fully understanding the position of the research subject, including all nuances and shades of interpretation, that research can progress. Deductive research which fails to take account of the totality of the research subject's position, might well produce statistically significant results that can reasonably be generalized from a sample population to a parent population. It is, however, unlikely to be predictive, as it has not taken account of subtle nuances that influence behaviour in the real world. Quantitative researchers counter this argument by attempting to incorporate more and more of these subtle nuances into their data collection in the form of variables. Qualitative researchers point to the mass of data this type of research generates and argue that theory testing frequently gets lost among a proliferation of confounding variables.

In contrast to quantitative research, qualitative research does not set out to test theory. Rather, it adopts an inductive approach which aims to develop a theoretical explanation about the social world under examination. In its extreme form it is not concerned with generalization, arguing instead that the theoretical explanation developed is bounded by the context within which the research took place (Halfpenny, 1979). The strength of this approach is seen to lie not in the predictive value of the research but in the increased understanding of the social world produced as a result of the analysis. A central issue for qualitative research is, therefore, the authenticity of the analysis. This in turn rests on the interpretation given to the data by the researcher. This position does, however, give rise to a central tension in qualitative research between an accurate and authentic portrayal of the research subject's world and the interpretation of this world by the researcher. Moerman (1974), a cognitive anthropologist, succinctly sums up this difficulty when he suggests that the use of the naive question from the 'outsider' researcher frequently relates to issues which are, from the natives' point of view, obvious or non-existent. Therefore, Moerman suggests, answering the researcher's question forces the actor to use categorizations that may not reflect their normal descriptions. Consequently the analysis produced cannot be said to reflect the normal meanings attached to behaviour by the actor. Similarly, Hammersley and Atkinson (1983) argue that qualitative researchers cannot simultaneously acknowledge the dynamic interactive aspects of the social world while at the same time denying the impact of interaction with the researcher upon that world.

Strauss and Corbin (1990), in addressing this issue, suggest that in order to authentically represent the social world qualitative researchers must render it 'anthropologically strange'. In other words, they must attempt to rid themselves of cultural baggage that may colour their interpretation of behaviour or responses given at interview. This is very similar to Garfinkel's (1967) idea of the naive question. Garfinkel argues that it is precisely the researcher's ability to ask naive questions that enables them to uncover culturally defined meanings or taken-for-granted assumptions which underpin behaviour but are so familiar to the respondents that they have ceased to notice them. In fact, as discussed in Chapter 1, a central concern for qualitative research is the problem of 'going native' or identifying so closely with the participants that it is no longer possible to adopt the detached stance regarded as necessary in order to articulate the principles underlying the observation of human action.

The concern with 'going native' or, alternatively, entering the research field with preconceived ideas, has been a central problem for qualitative research. This has led Glaser and Strauss (1967) to argue against even doing a literature search before commencing data collection, as they fear that the findings of previous research may colour and distort the qualitative research process. Bryman (1988) has provided a succinct analysis of the difficulties of adopting this position in any research project. He points out that all researchers approach research topics with some preconceived ideas about the nature of the subject under study, even if this only derives from their reasons for conducting the study in the first place. Reading literature about the subject is no more likely to contaminate the research process than knowledge gained from other, possibly less rigorous sources.

QUALITATIVE RESEARCH, NURSING AND
PRACTITIONER RESEARCH

A number of writers have highlighted the sympathetic relationship that appears to exist between qualitative research and the development of women's knowledge (Bowles and Klein, 1983; Smith, 1988). Part of the argument rests on the failure of a predominantly male research tradition to even identify issues of gender and gender-dependent knowledge in their research protocols and hypothesis testing. Thus a large area of human experience is rendered invisible (Smith 1988). Other writers have aligned male gender traits of control and prediction with the epistemology of quantitative research, and the female gender traits of nurture and understanding with the epistemology of qualitative research (Daly and Caputi, 1987). Whatever the reasons, it appears that nursing, which is a predominantly female occupation, seems to have developed an intuitively sympathetic stance towards qualitative research (Melia, 1984; Leininger, 1985).

A central strength derived from the process of rendering qualitative data as 'anthropologically strange' rests on the non-judgemental stance associated with mainstream anthropological research. The aim of such research is to understand cultures but not to judge them. Judgement implies the imposition of a preordained value system which, if used to analyse the data, would produce a deductive analysis. This is because the underlying culture would be interpreted according to the value system imposed on the data by the researcher. Consequently, the value system of the culture under study would never be fully extrapolated and understood.

Although these ideas have been warmly received in nursing, on closer examination their unqualified adoption would seem to be problematic for nurses. The difficulty arises from the premise that the authenticity of the analysis rests on the adoption of a 'naive stance' towards the collection of data about nurses. This suggests that it is much more difficult for nurses to undertake research into nursing practice than for others (e.g. sociologists) to do so, as the socialization process experienced during practice would make it very difficult for the nurse researcher to cultivate a naive stance towards data. However, if, as argued in Chapter 1, we accept that nurses undertake research into nursing practice for different reasons and to fulfil different aims from social scientists, then the process of data collection and analysis must be realigned to accommodate the different aims of the research.

It was suggested in Chapter 1 that most nurses undertake research into practice in order to improve it. The research therefore has an instrumental aim that is not usually found in social science research. It follows, therefore, that when nurses research practice it is not the world of their nursing colleagues that they primarily wish to study, but that this is only of interest in so far as it sheds light on another world, the world of practice and, more importantly, practice knowledge.

SOCIAL SCIENCE VALIDITY AND PROFESSIONAL KNOWLEDGE: CONTRADICTORY PERSPECTIVES

The world of nursing research has been dogged by prescriptive value-laden interpretations of research findings. Even if the nurse researcher conscientiously manages to remove all trace of judgemental or prescriptive interpretations from their data analysis, once it is published colleagues will not be so kind. The published research will invariably be interpreted through the value-laden lens of the professional aspirations of the reader.

If we take Melia's (1984) classic study of the professional socialization of student nurses, it is apparent that she went to great lengths to adopt a non-judgemental stance towards the data. She even wrote up the study as a book within the framework of a sociological analysis of work (Melia, 1987), rather than a partisan analysis of professional socialization. Others are not so patient. Nurses reading Melia's work will argue strongly that it provides substantive evidence that the two worlds experienced by student nurses during training, *should* be integrated. Immediately a prescriptive value-laden interpretation overrides the careful non-judgemental stance adopted by the researcher.

Values, it would appear, are the cornerstone of professional knowledge and of professional aspirations. For research to deny the existence of such values is in many ways to deny a political reality. Moreover, numerous research projects take for granted a professional perspective and consequently set out value-laden aims. For instance, projects may take for granted the superiority of primary nursing over team nursing or task allocation; or they may start from the assumption that the nursing process is a better method of planning care than the traditional kardex system. In each case the assumptions underpinning these projects have a strong professional rationale and can be justified from a professional perspective. However, they cannot simultaneously claim to be value-free or non-judgemental; on the contrary, they are laden with professional values.

The above discussion seems to highlight three issues: the first is the difficulty experienced by nurse researchers using qualitative research to render the data anthropologically strange for the purpose of analysis. The second is the use made of the findings: even if the nurse researcher succeeds in adopting a non-judgemental approach to data analysis, the profession rarely does. The third is the aims of professional research, which are not coterminous with the aims of social science research, seeking instead to increase professional knowledge.

Given the pervasiveness of these issues in setting the agenda for nursing research, it would appear incumbent upon nurse researchers to accept their implications for their research, rather than continue to deny them. So what are the implications for nursing research?

First, it follows that in seeking to further the professional aims of nursing, nurse researchers cannot simultaneously claim to undertake inductive research, even if they use qualitative methods of data collection. The adoption of a professional perspective means that nursing actions recorded during the course of data collection are interpreted according the dictates of this perspective. If researchers are not careful, they can fall into the trap of adopting the moral high ground. This can give rise to discussions of the data in terms of 'good' or 'bad' practice. This happens even when the researcher attempts to avoid it, as they cannot control the subsequent use made of their findings by the various political lobbyists.

If this is the case, then it would appear sensible for nurse researchers to acknowledge this perspective from the beginning of the research. This means recognizing that any data collected will be interpreted by some 'in the best possible light' and by others 'in the worst possible light'. Given the difficulty nurse researchers face in rendering their data anthropologically strange, this can even happen within the data analysis itself.

This creates a number of difficulties for nursing research. For instance, an adverse interpretation of the data from a professional perspective, e.g. one that indicates that the nursing action did not meet acceptable standards of care, adopts a rather superior stance towards the data. It implies that others in similar circumstances could have done better. This may or may not be true, but certainly cannot be substantiated from the data. Equally, the adoption of an empathetic stance which attempts to interpret all nursing action in the best possible light is problematic as it fails to develop a critical discourse with practice.

Notions of good and bad practice are value judgements. Their introduction would appear to undermine the validity of the data analysis. Yet, as argued above, it is difficult for nurses undertaking research into practice to deny all prior knowledge and to remove the influence of this knowledge from their interpretation of the data. Moreover, to do so denies the professional agenda that distinguishes nursing research from other forms of research. It is possible to argue that to deny the professional agenda will ultimately curtail the development of professional knowledge. This is because, from the perspective of social science, the introduction of value judgements, which reflect the professional agenda, would render the research findings invalid. If findings that reflect the professional agenda are declared invalid by social science, then the knowledge needed to underpin this agenda can never be forthcoming.

PROFESSIONAL VALIDITY AND PROFESSIONAL KNOWLEDGE: A SYNTHESIS

It was argued above that the professional agenda negates the possibility of undertaking inductive research, as all data analysis will be filtered through the lens of professional aspirations and coloured by notions of 'good' and 'bad' practice. If, and only if, this is accepted as the case, it follows that the professional agenda, loaded as it is with notions of 'good' and 'bad' practice, should be recognized and made explicit from the beginning of the research, and used to inform both the design of the research and the subsequent analysis of the data. For instance, depending on the type of research being undertaken, it may be possible to use professional values as a framework for both data collection and data analysis. Although this appears to adopt a deductive approach to data collection, it is in fact possible to use the framework as a heuristic device for both interrogating practice and testing out the values contained within the framework.

In my own research this was achieved by developing a professional framework which reflected the aims of care for high-, medium- and low-dependency patients. The framework was derived using a modified Delphi survey technique (Procter and Hunt, 1994) and identified aims of care for selected activities of living for such patients. During the observation stage of the research, patients were assessed and categorized according to dependency. The aims of care for the respective dependency category, derived from the modified Delphi survey, were given to the nurses, who were asked to identify which, if any, aims applied to a particular patient. Once the nurses had identified relevant aims they were asked to specify how, if at all, they intended to meet these aims during the forthcoming shift. The care given was observed and, time permitting, discussed with the nurses at the end of the shift.

In retrospect, it seems likely that the aims of care derived from the modified Delphi survey could have been obtained from a synthesis of nursing models or distilled from a meta-analysis of research findings. The decision to undertake a Delphi survey highlighted the importance that my supervisor, Maura Hunt, and I attached to articulating the value system and aims of care as defined by experienced practising nurses. The respondents in the Delphi survey were all ward sisters/charge nurses, chosen because we felt that their grade denoted both experience and a responsibility for identifying and meeting patient care needs within the ward environment.

Using this group of staff also grounded the findings in the realities of practice. This was considered to be important, as we felt that nursing models and research frequently fail to take account of both the context and complexities of practice (Hunt, 1987). This is because they tend to reflect the concerns of the underlying academic discipline which acts deductively as a source of knowledge for the development of the nursing model or research finding. It followed that a research framework derived from either of these sources might not be feasible within the constraints of a busy ward. A framework derived from practising nurses might also be problematic as it was essentially idealized – however, it would at least reflect the professional aspirations of this important group of staff.

Using this methodology allowed for an integration between theory, as espoused in the findings of the modified Delphi survey, and practice as observed on the ward. However, it avoided the prescriptive imposition of theory on to practice associated with traditional notions of deductive research. It did this by entering into a dialogue with the nursing staff which enabled them first to identify and secondly to define the criteria contained in the Delphi framework that they felt were relevant to their practice. It was perfectly possible for the nurses to reject all the criteria, or to introduce additional criteria, although this did not actually happen.

The approach described facilitated the development of a reflexive dialectical collection and analysis of data that closely resembles the process of analysis described by Winter (1987). As Winter suggests: 'Action research thus proposes a move "beyond" theories (whether mundane or academic) which prescribe and justify an interpretative basis for action towards a reflexive awareness of the dialectic between such theory and action, a dialectic which can sustain their mutuality while *transforming* both' (Winter, 1987, p.150), (Winter's underlining, my italics).

The issue of transformation became central to my notion of data collection and analysis, although in this case I did not set out to transform or change nursing action or behaviour, partly because I had no grounds for doing so, but also because the study was initiated by a Regional Health Authority and not the nurses whose practices I was privileged to observe. What I was able to do, however, was transform the theoretical notions outlined in the Delphi survey into concrete manifestations of nursing practice. Simultaneously I was also able to transform mundane practice into theory, regardless of whether the practice was reflected in the definition of nursing produced by the modified Delphi survey or fell outside this definition. Nursing action which fell outside the definition produced by the modified Delphi survey was not rejected or defined as either good or bad practice, but used to highlight the contradictions and complexities which are an everyday aspect of practice rarely captured adequately in theory.

For instance, I found that qualified nurses were frequently observed to take decisions in areas traditionally regarded as the province of medical staff, such as adjusting intravenous–venous fluid intakes, initiating oxygen therapy and referring patients to physiotherapy, occupational therapy or other professions allied to medicine. In every case they informed the medical staff of their actions, but were not observed to have the initial decision ratified by the doctor before implementing it. This finding can be contrasted with the difficulties qualified staff experienced in altering the implementation of care in relation to nursing needs. The aims of care identified in the framework emphasized nursing care and not medical care. However, in practice qualified staff exercised greater autonomy in the realm of medical care than nursing care. This finding required a modification of the analysis of nursing work to accommodate this apparent contradiction.

Using this method it was possible to simultaneously embrace both a deductive approach and qualitative inductive approach to the research. The development of the framework, although inductively derived from the Delphi survey, became deductive during the observation stage of the research. Here, it clearly identified the parameters of the professional agenda and used these parameters to structure both the collection and the analysis of data during interviews and observation. To this extent, therefore, it imposed an externally derived framework on to the analysis of the nurses' work. It therefore clearly did not conform to the tenets of qualitative research as set out by proponents such as Halfpenny (1979). It did, however, reflect approaches to research that have sought to mix, or in some cases integrate, qualitative and quantitative approaches within one research project. Bullock, Little and Millham (1992) discuss the advantages and difficulties of this approach in social policy research. Indeed, as the authors indicate, the mixing of methods seems to be a common feature of social policy research, perhaps because, like nursing, the research is not simply about understanding the social world but also about transforming it.

Bullock, Little and Millham (1992) highlight the importance of using theory to inform the development of research questions and the subsequent collection and analysis of data. They used the idea of 'process and career' or 'career routes' as a conceptual framework for investigating and developing explanations as to why family links declined over time for children in care. This concept was chosen from a number of potentially relevant theoretical constructs to inform the research process from the beginning. Clearly, had they chosen another framework the outcomes of the research would have been very different, but as people experienced in and knowledgeable about the field, it appeared to be a strong starting point.

The strength of this approach, as highlighted by Bullock, Little and Millham (1992), is that it allows theories generated from previous research findings to be used and refined in different situations. It therefore introduces a cumulative element to research, which is glaringly absent from purist approaches to inductive research. This can be justified in applied disciplines such as social policy and nursing, which are unlikely to progress their knowledge base unless they are able to engage in this process. Bullock, Little and Millham conclude by suggesting that rather than adopting, from a philosophical perspective, either a quantitative or a qualitative research method, researchers should begin with a theoretical formulation of the issue and then choose an appropriate method. As their study illustrates, adopting a theoretical formulation of the problem does not rule out the subsequent use of qualitative methods of data analysis, as implied by classic interpretations of qualitative methodology.

In my own research the values embedded in the professional definition of nursing, developed from the modified Delphi survey, provided the theoretical constructs used in the subsequent collection and analysis of data. More importantly, perhaps, it sparked off a tremendous debate with the ward nurses whose practice was being observed. This debate centred on the validity of the aims in relation to the professional agenda of nursing, and the translation of these aims into practice. Traditional qualitative researchers might object to the introduction of a deductive framework in what claims to be qualitative research, arguing that it distorts the reality of practice as it is experienced by nurses and patients on the wards. However, this is only an issue if the ward is an object of research and not the subject. In other words, the ward becomes an *object* of research when it is defined as a subculture and nursing practice is explored as an interesting manifestation of human action. If, as is argued in Chapter 1, practitioner research views practice as the *subject* of research, and aims to further practice knowledge, then it cannot simply stop at an analysis of action. It must explore the impact of that action on the concern of the practitioner, i.e. on patient care and, in particular, an improvement in that care.

The framework therefore became the medium for interrogating practice as, for the purposes of the research, it is within the framework that the professional knowledge resides. This means that observations of nursing practice are used to validate the framework as a tool for developing nursing knowledge. Practice, however, remains central to the data analysis. Adopting a qualitative approach to data collection means that aspects of practice not accounted for in the framework cannot be ignored, as can happen when the research is quantitative. Therefore, practice which does not conform to the framework is not necessarily discounted; rather the framework is found to be lacking because it is unable to account for the realities of practice as observed during the data collection. This rests on the notion that practice is, in the final analysis, real and that the realities of practice in all its manifestations cannot be denied or overwritten by a purely theoretical framework. Changes must occur in the framework to accommodate the complex dimensions of practice and not the other way round. The following example, taken from the data collection, illustrates the point.

I was observing the care being given on a traditional long-stay care of the elderly ward. The ward was based on the Nightingale design and had not been modified to meet the specialized needs of this care group. The early shift started at 7.30 a.m., and breakfast arrived at 8.30 a.m. It was served out by the domestic staff to patients who were sitting by their beds. Most of the patients required considerable help in getting up, toileting, washing and dressing before breakfast. An explanation as to why it was necessary to complete this care on all patients prior to breakfast being served has been written elsewhere (Procter, 1989a). The first hour was therefore very hectic. As usual, used commodes piled up in the middle of the ward as the nurses strove to complete the care required by the patients prior to the arrival of breakfast. On one occasion the following incident was observed. A student nurse came out from behind the curtains where she had been assisting a patient to get dressed. She saw the breakfast trolley advancing down the ward. She saw the commodes piled up in the middle of the ward and then she saw an elderly patient wander out from behind another set of curtains. This patient was half dressed and was searching for the rest of her clothes. It was apparent to me as a nurse observer that the student was faced with a dilemma – did she remove the commodes to the sluice, as it is unsavoury for patients to eat breakfast in close proximity to them, or did she attend to the needs of the wandering elderly patient? Both were urgent. The choice made by the student was not really an issue for nursing research, although it might be for a sociologist, as it would highlight definitions, priorities and values. From a nursing perspective what was interesting was that the situation arose at all. The juxtaposition of the situation becomes data in relation to a framework of nursing aims, regardless of whether or how the problem is solved or not in practice. In other words, I used my own professional knowledge and expertise to identify a dilemma that confronted a nurse during the course of her practice, regardless of whether or not she was aware of this dilemma. The identification of the dilemma was validated by the aims of care contained in the framework, which highlighted both the need to maintain patient dignity and the need to promote nutrition. I witnessed a situation where both could not be maintained simultaneously. This approach, therefore, highlighted the problematic nature of practice. It turned a dense but flat surface analysis of practice into a many-layered analysis that does not rest exclusively on an interpretation of behaviour (i.e. which need did the nurse choose to meet, and why?) but rather rests on a tension between the validity of the framework versus the validity of action. Using this approach action is only interesting insofar as it tells us something about the nature of nursing work, as exemplified in the framework. This could be:

- A deficit in the framework;
- A contradiction in the framework;

- An overinclusive framework;
- A theoretical development of the framework.

In many ways this approach is similar to positivist notions of the experiment. If we return to the description of quantitative research given at the beginning of this chapter, it is apparent that in quantitative research the variables to be considered in the research are predetermined by the researcher, regardless of whether they are considered relevant by the respondent. Using a framework, as described above, is in many ways doing a very similar thing, i.e. predetermining what is relevant for an analysis of practice. To this extent it reflects quantitative deductive notions of research.

However, it can also be used to generate dialogue with the practitioners. For instance, in the above example the framework of practice used during the research contained the two values of patient dignity and the need for an appropriate environment for consuming food (among other values). This had already been discussed with the student nurse prior to the observation of the above episode. The framework asked the nurse to identify the aims she thought were important in relation to nursing a specific patient on that ward. When I went back and looked at the framework she had completed she had highlighted both of these aims as important; she had also made the comment that it was often difficult to achieve on this ward.

The importance of this is not that it validates my interpretation of the dilemma facing the nurse: my own professional judgement was sufficient for that. The importance lies in the dialogue it generates with the nurses. The fact that this nurse had highlighted the importance of both values meant that I could conclude that non-attendance to one or other of the situations did not arise out of ignorance of the need for care: important in a situation where nursing care deficits are frequently observed and attributed to a lack of care on the part of the nursing staff.

Using the framework to generate a dialogue with the nurses about their definitions of care has a number of advantages. One such advantage is that it allows for the nurses' definitions and meanings of practice to be included in the analysis and juxtaposed against the definition of care contained in the framework. To this extent, then, the research is inductive as, unlike with traditional positivist research, the researcher is interested to know what the nurses think about the framework, whether it is relevant to their practice, whether there are gaps or contradictions. These questions are open-ended and therefore resemble the qualitative questions asked in semistructured interviews. The nurses' responses to the questions are used to modify or develop the framework according to the nurses' interpretation of practice.

From discussions with the nurses it was apparent that they attached great importance to the aims of care outlined in the framework. They went to great lengths to convince me, as the researcher, that they fully supported the aims of care given in the framework and highlighted their relevance for the patients on the ward. They did not seem unfamiliar with the language of the aims, even though this was abstract and non-specific. Evidence for this was found in their ability to operationalize abstract aims identified as relevant for individual patients. There was, however, a tendency to circumscribe the selection of relevant aims of care for individual patients to those that could be achieved within the prevailing ward routine. The subsequent operationalizing of each of the aims for a specific patient also tended to reflect the routine.

This data were particularly interesting as they highlighted how nurses rationalized the provision of routine care within a professional agenda of nursing aims. It therefore facilitated generalizations of the research findings from the micro-situation of the practice setting to the macro-agenda of professional aspirations, which informed the framework in the first place. This was achieved because, using the framework, the nurses were able to articulate the connection between mundane nursing practices such as feeding, washing or mobilizing patients and theoretical constructs such as independence and dignity outlined in the aims of care for specific activities of living given in the framework. Bridging the gap between theoretical formulations of practice and the realities of practice would appear to be an extremely important development for validating professional knowledge, and a considerable strength of this particular approach.

Further evidence of this process was found in the numerous contradictions that emerged when the nurses attempted to implement all of the aims of care they identified as relevant for a given patient. For instance, contradictions were highlighted between maintaining hygiene and promoting independence in patients who were incontinent. Nurses recognized the importance of encouraging patients to wash themselves, but were concerned about the effects on skin integrity if the wash was inadequate. A similar problem arose in relation to feeding patients. If nurses encouraged patients to feed themselves, the process took so long that the food became cold, congealed and unpalatable. Nurses commented on these contradictions as they attempted to operationalize divergent aims of care (such as 'promote independence' and 'ensure adequate nutritional intake') found in relation to specific activities of living.

Using this approach to data collection meant that even within the fairly narrow and circumscribed definition of nursing needs produced by adherence to the ward routine, contradictions in meeting the care needs of patients became apparent. Although it is not possible to be certain, I felt that such contradictions would have been difficult to generate without recourse to the aims of care given in the Delphi framework. Moreover, the nurses' attempts to operationalize divergent aims of care made visible the contradictions in those aims. Once the contradictions were highlighted it was possible to observe the process by which these contradictions were resolved within the ward setting.

The process of data collection and analysis described above was useful as it ruled out ignorance or lack of education as an explanation for any deficits in the care observed. Instead, it forced me to identify other explanations, which arose partly from contradictions between aims which only become manifest in practice and partly from structural constraints such as skills mix, staffing levels, equipment and ward design (Procter, 1989b).

The process by which this analysis was produced very much reflects the dialectical process described by Winter (1987). As Winter suggests, the strength of action research lies in the fact it does not use theory merely to explain action. Rather, it subjects the theories to a critical analysis of their 'locatedness' (Winter, 1987, p.150), or appropriateness within the practices of those whom the theory was developed to serve. It follows that a study that sets out to develop a critical analysis of the relevance of a theory for practice must first identify its theory. Having done so does not necessarily mean that the subsequent research has to adopt a quantitative methodology. This would imply the search for a causal analysis. In none of the research projects described in this chapter was causal analysis an aim. All of the research projects described sought to uncover meaning and identify relevance. In my case I sought to uncover the meaning and relevance of theoretical nursing constructs such as dignity and independence through a critical analysis of their relevance for the nurses in the study and the possibility of realizing these aims in the everyday world of nursing practice.

Finally, the mixing of deductive and inductive approaches to research, described above, facilitates the development of a cumulative body of knowledge without resorting to the restrictions of a deductive, quantitative approach to theory testing. A framework that incorporates professional values can be tested and modified in one situation and then tested again in a different situation. This becomes acceptable once it is acknowledged that nursing research is about developing a professional knowledge base. It is not about understanding the culture of nursing. Qualitative research methods can be used to develop this knowledge, but the validity of the analysis will reside in the increased understanding about practice that arises from the research as a result of developing or testing a framework that incorporates this knowledge base. Once this approach has been adopted, it is important to recognize the strength of traditional approaches to qualitative research and not reject information given by nurses because it does not conform to the framework. At the end of the day, validity resides in practice and not in the framework. A true test of the validity of the research would be in the fashioning of the framework to meet the needs of practice.

CONCLUSION

This chapter has highlighted some of the issues confronting nurses who want to undertake research into their own practice using qualitative research methods. It has revisited the debate about qualitative and quantitative research methods and discussed the difficulty confronting nurses when they attempt to adopt a naive, non-partisan stance towards data collection and analysis using qualitative research methods. The discussion develops the debate introduced in Chapter 1 about the aims of practitioner research and recognizes the emphasis on improving care which frequently predominates. Once it is recognized that practitioner research sets out to improve care, not merely to study it, then it becomes possible to reformulate traditional notions of validity in qualitative research to reflect this aim.

It is argued that the notion of improving care is derived from a concern to promote a professional agenda or the professional values of nursing and that these values are likely to influence not only the aim of the research but also the data collection, analysis and subsequent interpretation of the research. Under these circumstances it is important that these values are made explicit from the beginning and used openly to inform each stage of the research process. In the example described in this chapter, a framework which reflected professional aims of care for activities of living for high-, medium- and low-dependency patients was developed. This was used to structure the collection and analysis of data collected using participant observation. The advantage of this approach was that it made the values underlying the research open and explicit. For the nurses whose practice was being observed, it provided the criteria against which their practice was going to be analysed. It enabled them to criticize the value system and to justify any departures in their practice from the aims of care as defined in the framework. This process made it possible to refine the framework to reflect the concerns and experiences of practising nurses. It enabled them to identify priorities in relation to the framework and to identify those aims of care which they felt were not applicable to their work situation.

This approach also enabled the researcher to take a non-judgemental stance towards the nurses' practice, as judgements were made in relation to the adequacy of the framework to reflect the concerns and realities of practice as experienced by the nurses. This last point is very important, as it shifts the emphasis in analysis from an interpretation of behaviour to a development of professional knowledge through refining the instruments used to construct that knowledge. It is anticipated that this instrument could be a nursing model or a new method of organizing the provision of care such as primary nursing or case management.

The disadvantage of such an approach for many nurse researchers is that it appears to impose a deductive framework on to practice, which appears to be contrary to many of the most cherished ideals of inductive qualitative research. However, it is not dissimilar to developments in feminist methodology and new-paradigm research, both of which openly acknowledge the difficulties inherent in attempting to undertake a 'value-free' analysis of qualitative data. Both feminist research and new-paradigm research attempt to overcome this problem by entering into a collaborative democratic relationship with the research subject. However, this is not without its problems. First, research subjects may not want such a relationship with the researcher. Second, the question as to who owns the knowledge generated in the research does not appear to have been adequately resolved. Finally, the problem of generalization within feminist and new-paradigm research also requires further development. Generalization implies that the research must be analysed at a sufficiently abstract level to be transferable to a different setting. It is not at all clear how this is achieved within a collaborative, democratic relationship. If it is achieved, the researcher's role appears to be that of facilitator, as presumably the research subjects have the analytical skills necessary to undertake the research for themselves, should they so wish.

The approach to research outlined in this chapter recognizes the need to share the value system that informs the research process with the research subjects. However, the emphasis is on the development of professional knowledge by entering a dialogue with practitioners and observing their practice. This method allows the researcher to refine the instruments used to construct professional knowledge, by testing out the instruments containing the knowledge in the much more complex world of practice and accepting that in the final analysis it is practice that must fashion the development of the instrument and not the other way round.

It is possible that this approach could lead to the development of cumulative knowledge about aspects of practice. This is important, as the development of cumulative knowledge is part of the maturation process of a discipline. The adoption of qualitative research methods may have hampered nurses in their quest to develop their own knowledge base because of the problems associated with generalization in qualitative research. However, as many nurses have argued (Webb, 1984), quantitative methods are unlikely to provide appropriate means for investigating the complexities of human action found in nursing practice. The approach outlined in this chapter appears to provide one possible way of overcoming these problems. It incorporates a deductive element, essential to replication, which underpins the process of generalization but tests out the generalized knowledge using a qualitative analytical approach which both respects and incorporates the views of the nurses and uses both the views of the nurses and their behaviour to refine and develop the knowledge base of practice as constructed in the deductive theory.

REFERENCES

Bowles, G. and Klein, R. D. (eds) (1983) *Theories of Women's Studies*, Routledge and Kegan Paul, London.

Bryman, A. (1988) *Quantity and Quality in Social Research*, Sage, London.

Bullock, R., Little, M. and Millham, S. (1992) The relationship between quantitative and qualitative approaches in social policy research, in *Mixing Methods: Qualitative and Quantitative Research*, (ed J. Brennan), Avebury, Aldershot.

Daly, M. and Caputi, J. (1987) *Webster's' First New Intergalactic Wickedary of the English Language*, Beacon Press, Boston.

de Vaus, D. A. (1986) *Surveys in Social Research*, George Allen and Unwin, London.

Garfinkel, H. (1967) *Studies in Ethnomethodology*, Prentice-Hall, New Jersey.

Glaser, B. G. and Strauss A. L. (1967) *The Discovery of Grounded Theory*, Aldine, Chicago.

Halfpenny, P. (1979) The analysis of qualitative data. *Sociological Review* ,**27**(4), 799.

Hammersley, M. and Atkinson, P. (1983) *Ethnography Principles in Practice*, Tavistock, London.

Hunt, M. (1987) The process of translating research findings into nursing practice. *Journal of Advanced Nursing*, **12**: 101.

Leininger, M. (1985) *Qualitative Research Methods in Nursing*, Grune and Stratton, New York.

Melia, K. (1984) Student nurses' construction of occupational socialisation. *Sociology of Health and Illness*, **6**(2), 132.

Melia, K. (1987) *Learning and Working: The Occupational Socialisation of Nurses*, Tavistock, London.

Moerman, M. (1974) *Accomplishing Ethnicity. Ethnomethodology*, Penguin, Harmondsworth.

Procter, S. (1989a) The functioning of nursing routines in the management of a transient workforce. *Journal of Advanced Nursing*, **14**, 180.

Procter, S. (1989b) *A Study of Effects on the Provision of Nursing Services of Dependence on a Learner Nurse Workforce to Staff Hospital Wards*, Unpublished PhD thesis, University of Northumbria at Newcastle.

Procter, S. and Hunt, M. (1994) Using the Delphi Survey Technique to develop a professional definition of nursing for analysing nursing workload. *Journal of Advanced Nursing*, **19**(5), 1003–81.

Silverman, D. (1985) *Qualitative Methodology and Sociology*, Gower, Aldershot.

Smith, D. (1988) *The Everyday World as Problematic*, Gower, Aldershot.

Strauss, A. and Corbin, J. (1990) *Basics of Qualitative Research*, Sage, London.

Webb, C. (1984) Feminist methodology in nursing research. *Journal of Advanced Nursing*, **9**: 249.

Winter, R. (1987) *Action Research and the Nature of Social Inquiry: Professional Innovation and Educational Work*, Gower, Aldershot.

Experiences of Practitioner Research

This section is composed of accounts of practitioner research projects, which have been chosen because we feel that they illustrate some of the problems and issues inherent in practitioner research. We asked the authors of these chapters to write as honestly as they felt able to about the problems that they had experienced. This has resulted in a number of the chapters in this section deviating from the traditional format of the research report; indeed, in some chapters the authors have abandoned it completely. This has probably arisen because the traditional research report, with its sections on literature, methods, analysis and results, has an inexorable momentum of its own – each section must follow on logically from the other, and diversion and doubt are not permitted. For those who wanted to write about their doubts and problems, there was great difficulty in combining this type of debate with an orthodox account of the study.

Some of the contributors identified this as an issue of confidence and personal development – indeed, for some the research was undertaken as part of a course, and was a first experience of substantial research. Feelings that the research was problematic were therefore attributed to incompetence on the part of the researcher, rather than inappropriateness on the part of the research method, and so there was a tendency to try to 'cover up' problems in case they were seen as evidence of inadequacy. Having had the opportunity to reflect on their study, some researchers have said that they would feel much happier about doing another project simply because they feel more confident about themselves as researchers – they realize now that the dilemmas that they experienced were resolvable through their own resources rather than by adherence to methodological textbooks.

For those who are simply interested in the results of the research described in these chapters, the experience of reading them may be disappointing. For those who are prepared to forgo the traditional research write-up in favour of a thoughtful and open account of the 'hidden' research process (the bit that does not appear in the write-up), then these chapters may well prove to be of interest.

PART TWO: A

Introduction

Both the chapters in this part describe research studies that reflect the tensions in practitioner research between quantitative and qualitative approaches and notions of objectivity and subjectivity. In Val Pirie's study there were conflicts between her role as a participant in the interactions that she studied and her role as an analyst of these interactions – conflicts which she saw as being between the 'subjective' experience of working with a child and the 'objective' demands of analysing that experience. For Chris Stevenson the tension between qualitative and quantitative approaches arose partly because of the predominant ideology of the organization that she worked in, which valued quantitative approaches to evaluation, her own undergraduate psychology education, which had emphasized a quantitative, experimental approach, and her more recent reading and developments, which had suggested that a qualitative, constructionist approach would be the most appropriate for her study.

Both Chris and Val attempt to combine qualitative and quantitative approaches within one study – an approach which, we are assured by many writers, is perfectly possible. That both experienced problems in doing so may well be a result of their lack of experience as researchers at the time they did their studies, but what is also apparent in both chapters is that the culture in which they worked pushed them in a particular direction – towards a quantitative approach. Not only was 'proper' research assumed to be quantitative in this culture, but it might well be the only type of research which is listened to or supported. In these circumstances the use of qualitative approaches needs to be defended very carefully, and confidence in qualitative methods is easily eroded.

CHAPTER 5

Researching into communicating with children – problems and issues of using a randomized controlled trial

Valerie Pirie

EDITORS' INTRODUCTION

The following chapter graphically highlights some of the issues that arise for practitioners undertaking research using an experimental design. Like most of the other research described in the book, this project aimed to improve practice. In medical research the clinical control trial has become the exemplary method for undertaking research designed to test for improvements in practice. It seems appropriate to use this method in any situation where a similar level of proof is required. In this case the practitioner (Val) worked in a Child and Family Psychiatry Unit and was interested in developing methods to improve communication between practitioners and the preschool children referred to the unit. She undertook a clinical control trial of preschool children in order to address the question of whether a hand puppet manipulated by a health care worker was more likely to elicit information from a child than would the health care worker alone?

The chapter raises a number of interesting issues in relation to practitioner research. As Val points out, it is difficult to know how far results obtained under experimental conditions can be generalized to the clinical situation. Ethical considerations prevented Val from including in the interview schedule highly sensitive questions that might be asked under normal clinical conditions. Moreover, the need to standardize the interview meant that Val felt unable to follow up, during the course of the interview, interesting responses from the children that would have been pursued under normal clinical conditions. It is apparent, therefore, that the experimental research design prevented the research from capturing the true complexity of the practitioner's work, leaving important areas of that work outside the research protocol.

Throughout the research Val was conscious of the fact she was pursuing two, at times incompatible, roles simultaneously. For instance, she found it difficult to maintain the researcher role during the interviews with the children, and occasionally she lapsed into a clinical role. She was also concerned that because she wanted the hand puppets to be effective in order to help with a difficult clinical problem she might inadvertently bias the research in favour of the puppets.

The research used resources and facilities available in the clinic, such as video equipment, a one-way mirror and a play sand tray. Although Val had the support of her colleagues for the research and for the use of these facilities, she still had to negotiate access to them on each occasion she wanted to use them. Each interview of a clinic client was timed to coincide with a visit by the child to the clinic for therapeutic purposes. Coordinating access to the necessary research equipment to coincide with the child's visit necessitated a considerable amount of liaison work. It was important, however, that the research did not create any unnecessary inconvenience to the parents or the child, as this could have had repercussions for their clinic care.

The use of videos also raised ethical issues. Normal research protocol suggests that the research videos are erased at the end of the research. In this case, however, videos also form part of the treatment of children, and under therapeutic conditions are kept as part of their records. A debate therefore arose as to whether videos of children attending the clinic, taken for research purposes, should be seen as contributing to the therapeutic process and maintained as part of the child's records. Again, this dilemma highlights the difficulties confronted by practitioners in separating their research role from their clinical role.

Finally, the research raises particularly interesting issues in relation to using an experimental design with small children. Developing research-based knowledge about appropriate communication strategies to use with preschool children is clearly an issue of great contemporary importance. If, however, the experimental method continues to have an exalted status in relation to issues of 'proof' and 'causality', certain areas of clinical practice could be rendered 'unresearchable' using this approach. Children present a case in point. While it might be possible to undertake a clinical control trial with children to test out a technological innovation, this becomes much more difficult when the innovation occurs in the realm of psychosocial intervention. Although Val was able to achieve a considerable level of compliance from the children, she did experience problems in attempting to standardize the interview procedure. These problems arose because the children responded differently to the interview situation. Some children were quite happy for their parents not to be present, whereas others would not let their parents and, sometimes, siblings leave the room.

Despite these problems, which could be stressful for everyone at times, the chapter is written in the detached style associated with this type of research protocol. Although Val clearly experienced considerable dilemmas and problems in conducting the research, these are not explored in depth in this chapter. Writing about feelings and results in the same chapter or article is difficult, but this seems to be particularly the case when the research methodology is derived from the classic experimental tradition. To write up an experiment or trial from a subjective point of view would negate any semblance of rigour essential to the traditional notions of validity applied to this method.

Overall this research presents some interesting observations. It provides a challenge to the use of the experimental design with small children in areas which could potentially unlock deep and sensitive issues. It highlights the limitations of the design as, for ethical reasons, it was not possible to ask sensitive questions that would normally have been pursued as part of the everyday practice of the clinician. At the end of the chapter Val questions whether the quality of the results produced was worth the effort involved in obtaining them. This seems to raise questions about the validity of the experimental method in relation to this area of practice. This does not, however, detract from the importance of the questions asked, and it clearly behoves researchers to rise to this challenge and develop appropriate methods that are both valid and sensitive to issues under discussion and the vulnerability of the client group.

INTRODUCTION

Central to my work as a nurse in a Child and Family Psychiatry Unit are the skills needed to communicate with children of all ages. An increased awareness of child abuse and the realization that great skill and sensitivity is required to interview children when abuse is suspected (Vizard and Tranter, 1988) has highlighted the importance of effective communication between professional workers and children. Such interviews are mainly undertaken by social workers and the police, but the knowledge and experience of health care workers also make an important contribution to the care of these children at all stages of the investigation and therapy.

Although publicity has given prominence to the need for specialized communication skills in the sphere of child abuse, there are numerous other situations where such skills are very important, particularly with younger children, and can significantly improve the quality of care given.

In the course of my work, I had become aware that there were very few guidelines available on communicating with preschool children, especially when some specific information is required from them. The 1989 Children Act stresses the importance of seeking children's views when significant decisions are being made about them. As I talked with colleagues, I realized that many felt unsure about how to approach young children effectively at such times. Everyone was also very aware of the need to make such interviews as unstressful as possible for the children.

A brief initial literature search suggested that this was an under-researched area, and I decided that I would like to look in a more formal way at the issue of interviewing preschool children. Practical restraints meant that my study had to be small and specific in its aims. My attention had been drawn to the use of puppets for interviewing children (Vizard and Tranter, 1988) and I was aware that we seemed to be using puppets increasingly within our unit. Most children seem to like puppets. They are seen as playthings and therefore familiar and 'safe'. They represent an ideal choice for situations where there is a need to facilitate conversation with a small child because talking with or through puppets is an essential aspect of playing with them – puppet games are rarely silent.

Although puppets have been recognized as a valuable aid in communicating with children, it is evident from the literature that their use in a therapeutic or imaginative context has not been subjected to systematic study. Most workers still rely on intuition and their own experience when using puppets with children. The questions I found myself asking were: Do puppets have a role to play in the interviewing of children? Can they be of use with all children or are there specific groups who are likely to benefit particularly, or not at all? Indeed might puppets sometimes be a hindrance? Can any child or health care worker with basic skills in communicating with children use puppets as an aid in interviewing, or are they best used in a specific way for which specialized training might be needed?

I decided to formulate a research question linking puppets with the interviewing of preschool children: Is a puppet manipulated by a health care worker more likely to elicit information from a preschool child than would the health care worker alone? I also decided that I would compare two groups: children attending a child psychiatry clinic and children from a local nursery school. I thought that children attending our clinic would have greater difficulty communicating with health care workers because of their emotional and behavioural problems. It seemed likely, therefore, that this group might benefit more from the use of puppets than would a group of children who had not been identified as having any particular emotional or behavioural problems.

It took some considerable time to reach this stage in the development of my project. I thought that in comparison to the hours of thinking and reading which had preceded the formulation of my 'simple' research question, devising and implementing the study design would be relatively straightforward.

Over the next few months, I was to learn that research with children in a clinical setting was not and perhaps never can be straightforward!

STUDY DESIGN – USE OF EXPERIMENTAL METHOD

My identified research problem related a particular action – the use or non-use of a puppet – with a specific outcome: the quantity and quality of communication with the child. The experimental approach, which allows a degree of control over extraneous variables, is a particularly suitable method for research which attempts to relate cause and effect. It seemed, therefore, to be the method of choice for my study. However, although the experimental approach is strong on internal validity, one of its drawbacks is that the results which are obtained may not then generalize to a real-life situation. For example, in the present study, although I attempted to simulate the conditions under which small children might be asked questions in a health setting, there were clearly a number of differences. Not least of these was the fact that I, as interviewer, knew that this was not a 'real' situation.

Another disadvantage of the experimental method, especially within the sphere of social research, is that some manipulation of the subjects is essential, however straightforward and innocuous the research problem and design may be. My study involved small children spending time with an unfamiliar adult, answering questions which they might find stressful and for purposes which were going to be of no immediate benefit to them. This manipulation of the subjects is, of course, an important ethical issue and is normally partially solved by explaining to potential subjects, in as much detail as the design allows, what is involved in the research, and they can then choose whether or not they participate. In my study such young children were involved that it was not possible for them to be approached directly, and so it was their parents who had to decide whether or not they were to participate.

I made every effort to ensure that the procedure was as pleasurable as possible for the children, and in fact modified it during the pilot study to reduce any possible stress. I stated that I would discontinue an interview if a child showed any signs of distress. I also felt that it was important that the parents should know that there was no 'hidden agenda': the research intentions were exactly as I described them.

RESEARCH PROCEDURE

Each child in the study was interviewed twice and before each interview
the child and parent would spend an introductory period in a playroom
(Figure 5.1). In the first interview I would begin by collecting basic
family information and then show the parent and child the equipment
and the interview room. After the parent had left I would introduce the
child to the puppet and begin the puppet interview. The second interview followed the same procedure, except that the puppet was not used
and that at the end the parent and child would watch the video of the
first interview.

The children in the sample were aged between 36 and 59 months, and
were selected from families referred to the child and family psychiatry
clinic where I work. The second group were recruited from a local
nursery school. I knew that young children would not be able to sit and
answer a series of questions, even on those occasions that the puppet
was involved, without something to play with – to have expected them
to do so would have been unfair. I therefore decided to interview them
while they were playing at a sand tray.

USE OF VIDEO

In order to collect as much data as possible on their verbal and non-
verbal responses, I needed to videorecord the sessions. This was done
through a one-way mirror and the children were aware that they were
being videoed. I originally intended that the parents would observe both
sessions through the one-way mirror, but during the pilot study parents
commented that they found it difficult not to discuss with the children
their responses to some of the questions, and this could of course affect
the child's response to the questions in the second interview. I therefore
decided to ask parents to observe only the second interview *in vivo* and
to view the first one from the videorecording. All parents agreed to this.
It is possible that the children's responses in the second interview were
affected because they knew that their parent was watching from behind
the one-way mirror, but I observed no obvious differences.

The only exception that was made to this procedure was when the
child refused to separate from the parent. The parent was then invited to
sit in the interview room with the child for both interviews, but was
asked not to discuss the child's responses before the second session.
There were only three children who would not separate from their
parent (two non-clinic boys and one clinic boy). Surprisingly, all three
children ignored the parent throughout the interview. In the case of one
of the non-clinic boys it was also necessary to include his younger sister

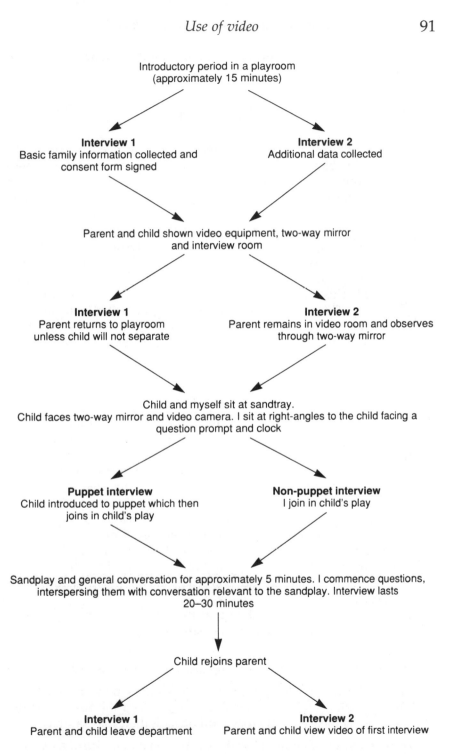

Introductory period in a playroom
(approximately 15 minutes)

Interview 1
Basic family information collected and
consent form signed

Interview 2
Additional data collected

Parent and child shown video equipment, two-way mirror
and interview room

Interview 1
Parent returns to playroom
unless child will not separate

Interview 2
Parent remains in video room and observes
through two-way mirror

Child and myself sit at sandtray.
Child faces two-way mirror and video camera. I sit at right-angles to the child facing a
question prompt and clock

Puppet interview
Child introduced to puppet which then
joins in child's play

Non-puppet interview
I join in child's play

Sandplay and general conversation for approximately 5 minutes. I commence questions,
interspersing them with conversation relevant to the sandplay. Interview lasts
20–30 minutes

Child rejoins parent

Interview 1
Parent and child leave department

Interview 2
Parent and child view video of first interview

Fig. 5.1 Research procedure.

in the session; she played quietly, and again it did not appear to affect the course of the interview.

STRUCTURE OF INTERVIEWS

In planning the research design I recognized the need to control for extraneous variables. I therefore intended that, as far as possible, every interview would be conducted in exactly the same way. After a short introduction, the children would be asked identically phrased questions in a set order, with minimal additional interaction between myself and the child. However, it was evident from the pilot interviews that the children found it quite stressful to be asked questions in this way. I therefore decided to relax the procedure and ask the questions more casually during the course of an extended interaction between myself and the child. This interaction related to the sandplay in which the child was involved. The phrasing and order of the questions remained the same, but there was considerably more variation in the length of the interviews and in the nature of the relationship which developed between myself and the child.

Questions used

The study aimed to investigate the use of puppets when asking children direct questions in a potentially stressful situation. I therefore had to compile a set of suitable questions and, since the children were to be interviewed on two occasions, I considered the possibility of developing two sets of questions so that they would not be subjected to the frustration of being asked the same questions twice. However, this would have necessitated a more complex crossover design and, given the small number of subjects involved, it was not feasible. I decided instead to leave a minimum of 2 weeks in between the two interviews, in the hope that this would minimize any frustration experienced by the children. One or two of the children did point out that they had already been asked particular questions.

The questions were planned so that the first four were very general and the content not thought to be stressful for small children, for example:

Can you tell me the names of everyone who lives in your house?

The next four were potentially more stressful, as they related to the children's relationship with their family and raised the issue of family members being pleased and cross with one another; for example:

Sometimes we do things which make our Mum and Dad pleased with us. What sorts of things do you do which make your Mum pleased with you?

The last two questions invited the children to ask or tell me or the puppet anything they liked. The questions appeared to be understood by most of the children, but were probably not entirely suitable for the children at the younger end of the age range. If the child failed to respond when the question was first asked, I repeated it only once and did not press the children to answer. Occasionally, if the child's response was unusual, particularly interesting or ambivalent, I spontaneously and unintentionally added a further prompt. In such instances I ignored any responses elicited by the additional prompt during the analysis of the videotapes.

ISSUES RELATING TO THE USE OF THE PUPPET

I gave considerable thought to choosing the puppet character which would be used in the project. Initially I decided to allow the children to choose from a range of puppets the one to which they would like to talk. However, during the exploratory stages of the research it became evident that it would be difficult for me to step into a series of different personae at short notice. Furthermore, the child might then be distracted by the other puppets and it would be more difficult to develop an appropriate introductory sequence. Therefore I chose an appealing polar bear puppet to use with all the children. I introduced him as my friend Polo and explained that he would like to play with the child.

Establishing the puppet persona proved much more difficult than I had expected. I made no attempt to acquire specialist puppetry skills, as most people using puppets in a health care setting would not be skilled in their use. It was difficult to find a suitable voice for Polo and eventually I just adopted a fairly high-pitched childlike voice. I made Polo male, without giving any consideration as to which gender would be most appropriate; it was only after the interviews had been completed that I noticed this oversight. I also presented him as younger than the children being interviewed, and not very clever or confident.

RESEARCHER BIAS

Practicality necessitated that I should also be the interviewer in this study. This raised the issue of bias, since I might have unintentionally given the children more positive cues in the puppet interviews and this might have encouraged a greater degree of response from them. I intended to assess the extent to which such bias affected the interviews by asking colleagues experienced in child work to rate the first 5 minutes of the interviews, asking them to rate the degree of effort they considered I had put into establishing a relationship with the child on a five-point scale, ranging from minimum to maximum.

A trial run of this rating exercise raised a number of problems:

- The raters had no baseline from which to rate my degree of effort.
- It was evident that there was an interactive effect between myself and the children and I was constantly adapting to the children's varying levels of responsiveness.
- Of necessity, I had to put more effort into the puppet interviews because of the need to play two roles, i.e. adult and Polo; furthermore, being Polo in itself demanded more effort since I had to create an appropriate character for him.

There did not appear to be any viable way of overcoming these fundamental difficulties, so I abandoned this exercise. However, although I did not manage to find an objective method of assessing the level of bias between the puppet and non-puppet interviews, I did notice that I felt much more relaxed in the non-puppet interviews. I found using the puppet quite difficult because of having to remember to maintain the puppet persona, and also because the children would often interact with me as adult at the same time as interacting with Polo, and there were times when I found it difficult to keep the boundaries between the two. My impression is that the fact that I was more relaxed during the non-puppet interviews may have counter-balanced any tendency to try and elicit more or longer responses from the children during the puppet interviews.

ANALYSING THE VIDEO TAPES

In order to do justice to the rich data generated by the videotaped interviews, I decided to analyse them both quantitatively and qualitatively.

Quantitative analysis

The quantitative analysis was intended to elicit data regarding the amount of information the children gave in the puppet versus non-puppet interviews. For this, I simply counted the number of words used in each child's response to each question and recorded the length of time taken by each interview.

I analysed the rate of looking and touching, as I thought these would be good indicators of the closeness of the relationship established between myself and/or the puppet and the child.

I used measures such as the number of times the child was distracted or tried to terminate the interview to determine whether the puppet increased the children's attention and concentration.

In order to maintain consistency in determining the above measures, I established a number of rules for the analysis of the videotapes. Mostly these were fairly straightforward, but counting the number of words in each response presented some problems because of inconsistencies in the way I asked the questions. In order to minimize the effects of my inconsistencies I made the following rules: that only responses to the first or second delivery of each question were counted; that responses to prompts which I gave inadvertently were not included; furthermore, if a child made an unrelated comment while answering a question this was not included as part of the response; and that repetitions of words while a child formulated an answer were not included.

Qualitative analysis

The qualitative analysis took the form of an account of some of the children's behaviours and responses which could not be quantified. This included the transcript of the complete interviews of one of the non-clinic children.

RESULTS

Rather disappointingly, and contrary to my expectations, the results of my study did not support my hypothesis that the children would respond more willingly and at greater length to questions asked by a puppet which is manipulated by a health care worker than to those asked by a health care worker alone. Nor was there any significant difference in their response to the puppet between the two groups of children.

The measures I used (the number of non-responses and the number of words used in response to the questions) indicated that there were no significant differences for either group between the puppet and non-puppet interviews. As there was also no interaction effect, my hypothesis that the clinic children would be more helped by the puppet was not supported by the data either. Although most children entered into a warm and more relaxed relationship with the puppet, treating him as a peer, this did not lead them to be more uninhibited or expansive in their responses. However, a significant difference did occur between the two interviews (puppet and non-puppet) in the number of responses from both groups, to the question: *What does your Dad do that makes you cross?* I thought this was probably the most stressful question which I asked the children because, even though they were so young, they may have felt that in responding to it they would be disloyal to their father. I was interested to note that the information the children gave to the puppet, but not to me, included responses such as 'shouting at me' and 'hitting me'. The responses given to this question suggest that children may be more willing to give sensitive information to a puppet rather than to an adult interviewer. However, on the basis of a single question this conclusion can only be tentative, and it would not be possible to explore this much further in a non-clinical interview as it would not be ethical to subject the children to many more stressful questions.

PROBLEMS RELATED TO BEING RESEARCHER AND PRACTITIONER

This study was carried out in the course of my normal work using the facilities in the department where I am employed. Practically, it would not have been possible for me to have sole use of the facilities for the time it would have required to have carried out the interviews in a block. I also had to arrange the interviews for the clinic children at times when they would normally be attending the clinic, so as not to inconvenience their parents unduly, and similarly find times that were convenient for the nursery children. This meant that over a period of several months I was regularly involved in clinical assessment and therapy sessions before and after the research interviews. This necessitated a constant switching between clinical and research approaches. Since my primary skills lie in the clinical area, I had to remind myself constantly that I must not stray outside the confines of the research design. This was particularly difficult when the child made an interesting comment which in a clinical setting I would have automatically tried to explore and develop further, but which the need for consistency within the experimental research approach could not allow. It was necessary to maintain this consistency so that a direct comparison could be made between the interviews, and so that quantitative analysis of the data could be carried out. However, almost certainly some interesting qualitative data were lost.

I found the planning and organizing of the research sessions stressful; I had constantly to check that the room and video facilities would be available and that the sand tray was not needed elsewhere. I had to ensure that the clinical work in the department was not being too affected by my frequent use of the facilities.

The use of video also created a serious problem at the planning stage, one which was really only resolved with a compromise. At the time that I was carrying out this study, it was departmental policy to regard all videorecordings made of the children as part of their clinical records. The clinicians responsible for the care of the children recognized that the videotapes were part of a research project and consequently not intended to be part of the children's assessment or therapy. However, because I worked as a member of the clinical team, and because the tapes would be made as part of the child's normal attendance at the department, it was felt that the tapes would have to be subject to the same conditions as non-research tapes. This meant that the tapes could not be erased, whereas normal research protocol would expect that they should be. In consultation with the department clinical team, I decided that the recordings made of the non-departmental children would be erased at the end of the research but that those made of children attending the department would be kept. Therefore, two different consent forms had to be used and parents of the clinic children were told that the recordings would become part of their child's medical records. Naturally, parents retained the right to refuse to have a videorecording made under these circumstances (the same right which they would have even if the tapes were not to be used for research purposes), and such a refusal would exclude the child from the project. In practice only two parents did not wish their child to participate in the project and in neither case was the videorecording stated as a reason for the refusal.

I also had to consider what action I should take if a child made any allegations of abuse during the interviews. I did not expect this to occur, as the questions I would ask were not intended to elicit such information. Furthermore, it seemed unlikely that a parent abusing their child, or aware that their child was being abused, would agree to take part in the project. However, I realized that there was a possibility that such information might be given, although unsolicited. I discussed this with the clinical team and we decided that should a disclosure occur in the course of an interview with a clinic child, I would follow the normal clinic procedures regarding allegations of abuse. The videorecording might then have to be used as evidence. If, however, the allegation was made by a non-clinic child, the tape would be erased as stated in the consent form, but I would ask the parent to take further action to ensure the safety of the child. This procedure would be in accordance with the ethical code of the Society for Research on Child Development, which states:

> When in the course of research, information comes to the investigator's attention that may seriously affect the child's well-being, the investigator has a responsibility to discuss the information with those expert in the field in order that the parents may arrange the necessary assistance for their child.
>
> (Rheingold, 1982, p.322)

In fact, no child made any such allegations.

I spent a great deal of time in the preparatory stages discussing the above issues with my colleagues and supervisor. It was very difficult trying to comply with both clinical and research procedures, and meant that this step in the research process was much more stressful than I had ever anticipated.

CONCLUSION

This project taught me a great deal about the research process and undoubtedly enhanced my ability to interview small children. I am pleased to have had the experience and welcome the personal gains. However, especially with hindsight, I do wonder whether the outcome justified the time and effort the design required. The video interviews took about 70 hours and the analyses probably longer.

It is difficult to know whether I achieved a level of objectivity compatible with an experimental approach. I suspect that my overriding priority that the children should in no way be stressed, together with the intrusion of my 'clinical' approach, made it impossible to keep the interviews consistent and that this may have affected the validity of the results. However, it was, of course, my involvement in clinical work and the realization of the very practical problems we faced that led me to this type of research rather than carrying out a something like a survey, which I think would have been much simpler and less stressful!

With thanks to Dr Brian Bell of the Institute of Health Sciences, University of Northumbria at Newcastle, for his help with this study.

REFERENCES

Rheingold, H. L. (1982) Ethics as an integral part of research in child development, in *Strategies and Techniques of Child Study*, (ed R. Vasta), Acedemic Press, New York, pp. 305–23.

Vizard, E. and Tranter, M. (1988) Helping children to describe experiences of child sexual abuse – a guide to practice, in *Child Sexual Abuse Within the Family: Assessment and Treatment*, (eds A. Bentovim, A. Elton, J. Hildebrand, M. Tranter and E. Vizard), John Wright, London, pp. 105–29.

CHAPTER 6

Reflections on evaluating a course of family therapy

Chris Stevenson

EDITORS' INTRODUCTION

This paper illustrates one of the issues facing practitioner research in health care today – the demands made on researchers that their data should produce 'objective' data which will fit with currently popular models of quality assurance and monitoring. Whereas it can be argued that asking practitioners to evaluate and monitor their practice is a healthy move which will stimulate development and change and avoid complacency, problems may arise in the potential conflict between researcher and organization about what constitutes 'valid knowledge'. Qualitative data, which to the practitioner captures the 'essence' of practice, may not be seen as rigorous or generalizable to managers, whereas the type of quantitative data which satisfies managers' demands may seem to the practitioner to be oversimplistic.

The debate may be seen as simply one of what constitutes valid knowledge, but it is perhaps better understood as a debate about the purposes that knowledge will be put to. For a manager, any study of a particular type of practice will be 'useful' in terms of how it helps them to do their job, which at its simplest will be to allocate resources or calculate costings, or to market the service. The manager will therefore want data about the 'effectiveness' of the service in terms of successful outcomes for the patient, along with figures about the costs involved in terms of staff time and resources. This type of data essentially simplifies the process of care, and packages it into a neat and tidy form. For the practitioner, however, the motivation for the study may come from a desire to know more about the process of care, the vagaries of different cases, the problems that may arise and the strategies that can be used, as well as the particular personal skills and qualities that the care requires. This type of knowledge is useful for developing a fine-grained analysis of care which will convey the experience to other practitioners so that they may learn from it, and in addition contribute to the professional skills of the researcher who carried out the study. In other words, the data from the study will be useful to the practitioner in the way that it helps the practitioner to do their job. It will therefore need to describe the complexity and messiness of the practice world.

Such descriptive research has credibility in some academic disciplines, such as nursing or sociology, although even here there have been furious debates about the 'scientific status' of qualitative approaches. It may be too soon to say that the battle for acceptance for qualitative research has been entirely won, but in general it is accepted in these disciplines as a valid mode of enquiry. In other disciplines, for example economics or management, and in the eyes of the general public, however, there is still a notion of 'proper research' as being essentially quantitative. This long-standing tradition puts the qualitative researcher at some disadvantage as they seek to defend their research against criticisms of subjectiveness, ironically often using positivist concepts in their defence. This is clearly apparent in this study, where Chris discusses the 'pull' of positivism, which came not only from her managers, but also from her experiences as a psychology student, where the experimental approach was paramount. This, Chris feels, led her at times to deny her position as insider, with all the subjective experiential knowledge this affords.

The dilemma for the practitioner who researches practice as a way of supporting the case for that practice with managers seems inevitable and insoluble. It is possible, of course, to argue that a practitioner should not advocate a practice for which there is no scientific evidence of its effectiveness, but this argument does little to explore the notion of what constitutes scientific evidence. Most practitioners will have experience of cases which did not behave according to scientific predictions, where scientifically approved treatment did not work, or where scientifically discredited approaches did. More commonly, there may be no scientific evidence available and the practitioner must work from experiential knowledge, theories-in-practice, or intuition, none of which have orthodox scientific status. This changes the argument from one about the necessity of scientific evidence to one about the nature of such evidence.

This debate is now being recognized in the theoretical literature on evaluation, and there is now a movement away from reliance on measurement towards more qualitative approaches (see, for example, Quinn Patton, 1988). These ideas, however, may take time to trickle down to managers who are working in the measurement-orientated culture of today's health services, and even longer to gain wide acceptance and support. In the meantime, the practitioner researcher who has to meet management and practice objectives is left trying to reconcile these two imperatives. Dividing the study into two parts, as Chris has done, may be the only practical solution, but it is one which creates its own problems, which the researcher would do well to be aware of.

INTRODUCTION

'Rabbit's clever,' said Pooh thoughtfully.
'Yes,' said Piglet, 'Rabbit's clever.'
'And he has Brain.'
'Yes,' said Piglet, 'Rabbit has Brain.'
There was a long silence.
'I suppose,' said Pooh, 'that that's why he never understands anything.'

(*The House at Pooh Corner*, A.A. Milne, 1928)

Birch (1987) argues that therapists 'just know' when they are doing good therapy and complicated theoretical attempts to understand it further may be misguided. However, in the context of developments in the NHS, which centre on the development of quality initiatives and consumerism, practitioners are encouraged to make systematic evaluations of their own practice to ensure that standards of effectiveness and efficiency are met in a 'less subjective' way than through therapist perceptions of success or failure. The dominant current model within the NHS is audit of practice. This is quantitative monitoring, i.e. how much of something goes on rather than what. For me, as a practitioner within an organization that favoured measurement-orientated quality assurance, there was the need to produce some quantitative figures, especially in relation to family treatment, which was a new facet of the service provided by the agency.

In addition, I felt the need as a practitioner to understand more about what happens in a course of family therapy. This was fuelled by two factors, first, my reading of evaluation research of the damage that can result from certain components of family therapy (Gurman and Kniskern, 1978). In particular, these authors emphasize the importance of therapist variables, especially 'relationship-building skills'. The importance of the latter is demonstrated by an anonymous reporter (1985) who gave a commentary on her family's experiences in therapy. The cursory introductions made by the therapist were followed by a rapid request that the family be videotaped. Her husband recalls that as he said, 'Okay', to the request, 'I pulled up my armour, locked it and threw away the key.' This suggested to me the need to explore the process of family therapy sessions in detail.

Closely linked to this was the need to develop further my own skills in working with families. Although I might 'just know' when I was doing good therapy, it seemed to me that through a close analysis of what happened as I did therapy I would gather some ideas of how I might adapt my approach to give families a better experience. In other words, I needed more specific feedback to fine-tune my approach.

The research therefore had to satisfy different demands placed upon it which informed the decision to develop an integrated quantitative and qualitative model of evaluation within a research/practitioner model. The quantitative aspect would fulfil agency requirements by providing data in a language that they understood, i.e. numbers, whereas the qualitative part of the study would inform me as a therapist about what happened when I engaged with the family in therapy. Parry, Shapiro and Firth (1986) strongly advocate the research practitioner model, suggesting that such a model can 'build a bridge between clinical realism and independent evidence'. This remark seems consistent with an approach that seeks to integrate quantitative and qualitative methods and with my need to gain feedback on my own practice.

THE STUDY

The study was within the context of a master's programme and directed by the needs discussed in the introduction above. The aims of the research were as follows:

- To evaluate the effectiveness of a family therapy team with a family using a single-case design and multiple quantitative outcome measures.
- To analyse the within-session therapeutic process, including immediate session outcome.
- To compare the within-session therapeutic process with the multiple outcome measures within the single-case design.

THE CONTEXT

I was fortunate in being a worker in a family therapy clinic within a community psychiatric nursing service. The clinic was run by myself and another family therapy worker, with additional supervision sought as necessary. Referrals for family work came from GPs, social workers and psychologists, but there was also a close enough relationship with these agencies for the family therapy workers to make a decision to convene a family when only the individual was identified initially as being in need of therapy. The clinic's way of working entailed families and the therapist being videoed in sessions, and a supervision team watching the therapy through a video link. This meant that there were few constraints on the research in practical terms, as I myself was the therapist and, with the family's permission, could simply use the videorecordings for process analysis.

The family chosen was referred to the service by a consultant psychiatrist who had seen the son, Peter, who was said to be 'classically depressed'. The psychiatrist highlighted Peter's closeness to the family – specifically his mother and father – as the last child still at home. He had failed his A levels and not gone to college as originally planned, but rather had been absorbed into the family business in the small town where the family lived.

The family attended for six sessions in all. They readily consented to take part in the research, which was framed as part of an audit process.

METHODOLOGY

The double design

For discussion purposes the design of the study can be conveniently divided into the quantitative and qualitative aspects, although issues around the integration will be discussed later.

Quantitative

The single-case design advocated by Hersen and Barlow (1976) was chosen in order to facilitate the gathering of detailed data. This involves looking at one case and taking frequent measures over time. Usually there is measurement of some symptom or behaviour during an assessment phase. This represents a baseline measure. By taking this initial measure, the individual becomes their own control, i.e. the baseline measure is seen as the 'no treatment' control measure which is found in random control trials. Following the assessment period, treatment is initiated and further measures are taken. Treatment is then withdrawn or a different treatment is begun. Repeated measurement over time allows a set of dependent measures to be generated which may then be analysed in terms of trends.

In this study, the single case used three measures:

- A measure of level of depression (Beck Depression Inventory (BDI), Beck *et al.*, 1961) in the person identified as the problem holder.
- A measure of the organization of the family (Bennun, 1986), developed from the Personal Questionnaire (PQ, Shapiro, 1961).
- A single measure of client satisfaction taken at the end of the course of therapy.

These first two measures were plotted over the course of the therapy.

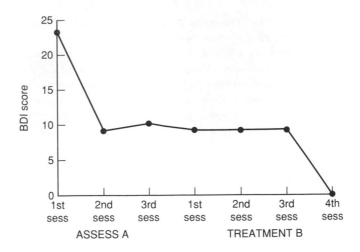

Fig. 6.1   Research procedure.

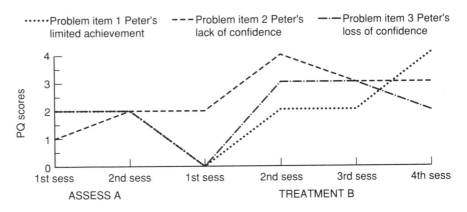

Fig. 6.2   Research procedure.

Figures 6.1 and 6.2 demonstrate the pattern of scores for the BDI and one item of the PQ to show the form of data generated. (As the purpose here is to reflect on the issues around the research rather than the work itself, the reader should refer to Stevenson (1993) for a full discussion of the research outcomes.)

At the end of treatment, the client satisfaction score was 1 on a scale of 1–5, with 1 as highly satisfied.

The quantitative measures indicated a positive outcome to therapy. The larger question remains of how far the single-case design is an appropriate means of evaluating practice.

CRITIQUE OF THE QUANTITATIVE STUDY

The single-case design has strengths and weaknesses:

- The design was easy to apply; it could feasibly be incorporated into all cases within an agency and so be used as part of clinical audit fitting the current NHS ethos.
- It generates the kind of data, i.e. numeric, which is valued and so sought by NHS management.
- As each case provides its own baseline, it avoids having 'no treatment' controls and so is ethically acceptable.
- There are no problems with comparisons between groups. Random control trials that claim groups are homogenous have been criticized (Frude, 1980).

There was some tension between being both a good researcher and a good practitioner through applying the single-case design. Although it was necessary to generate enough data for the quantitative analysis, there was a risk of losing the family by overburdening them with too many questionnaires. This was against my priority as a therapist of helping the client through a well defined treatment programme. Burnham (1986) has suggested that it is difficult to separate assessment and intervention as, for instance genograms as an assessment tool raise the family's awareness of dynamics.(Genograms are extended family trees which contain information about family roles and relationships.) Similarly, the PQ completed by the family focused on the family structure. Nevertheless, it felt to me that we were being distracted from the 'real' work of therapy. This issue is revisited later when the tensions of being an insider and outsider to the research area are debated.

Quantitative methods help us to know what happens but not why. In other words, the design generated data that allowed the therapy to be evaluated as effective and so fulfilled the agency requirement on the researcher to evaluate, but it did not in any way define what the therapist's role was within this. How far, then, did the decision to incorporate the qualitative aspect of the research address this point?

USING QUALITATIVE METHODS

Alongside the single case, I wanted to analyse what happened in my sessions with the family. This was to be the source of information as to why certain outcomes were found in the course of the therapy, as measured within the single-case design, and also to contribute to my understanding of my own practice.

Process study is a qualitative method which has been applied to clinical settings. Parry, Shapiro and Firth (1986) describe process study as the intensive analysis of the process of change, using language meaningful to the practitioner. Rather than using case reporting, or being driven by previously proposed theory, process study is rooted in evidence gathered through fine-grained analysis of the therapy sessions.

Qualitative data analysis brings its own problems. It presents data that are rich in content but vast in amount, leaving the researcher with the challenge of finding some system of meaningful organization. Within process study of psychotherapy frameworks do exist which have attempted to help structure the analysis of experiential therapy sessions. In this context, Greenberg (1986), drawing on the work of Elliott (1983), suggests that the focus of process study must be significant change events, i.e. an interactional sequence between the client and therapist, with a clear beginning and conclusion and which is likely to have a therapeutic effect. 'The event is like a short incident in a novel or drama', (Greenberg, 1984, p.138). Both therapist and client are able to recognize the change events. In any session there may be one or many of these change events, which are themselves divided into components (see Heatherington and Friedlander (1990) for a fuller description of Greenberg's schema). These components are a means of structuring the analysis of the change events.

However, the variables to be studied within the components of change events are not specified. For this reason, I carried out an initial pilot study to isolate those variables that seemed most applicable to family therapy. This was achieved through applying the principles of grounded theory. Glaser and Strauss (1967) developed grounded theory to help the discovery of theory embedded within large amounts of qualitative data. The researcher develops conceptual categories that fit the data. By looking within and between categories clear, consistent boundaries can be set up. The conceptual categories can then be linked and ultimately refined into some theoretical idea.

An example may make the procedure clearer. In looking at a change event the researcher would be interested in:

- What the family was doing in terms of resistance/compliance and alliances with each other and the therapist;
- What the therapist was doing in terms of technique, and where she was in relation to the family, i.e. whether she was in control or not;
- How the family responded to this in terms of their verbal behaviour and inferred non-verbal behaviour, e.g. whether family beliefs or myths are being challenged. (See Stevenson (1993) for a full account of the levels of process analysis and the associated variables.)

Following the pilot study, a ready-made framework consisting of a modified version of Greenberg's (1986) schema fleshed out with variables designated as important was adopted for the analysis of sessions in the main study. This framework applied to videoed therapy sessions allowed the identification of therapist and family 'behaviourial' sequences in the data.

CRITIQUE OF THE QUALITATIVE STUDY

I entered the research project as an 'insider' in ethnographic terms, that is, as a practitioner I was already party to the language, beliefs and everyday practice of the family therapy team. I was one of them. Woolgar (1993) describes ethnography as 'a sceptical descriptive analysis of the taken for granted'. However, it is difficult to maintain the distance required for analytical scepticism when you are an insider. This tension was most apparent in the process study. It was relatively easy to revert to being an 'outsider' in the quantitative part because the methods of data collection almost imposed distance and a greater degree of impartiality, although there was some tension around the multiple administration of questionnaires discussed above.

My insider position affected the way in which I 'discovered' variables from the data via grounded theory analysis. It was inevitable that the analysis was informed by my training and theoretical assumptions. Henwood and Pidgeon (1992) quote Feyeraband's (1975) assertion that legitimate data are necessarily defined through theory. Without this framework, '. . . what grounds grounded theory!' (Henwood and Pidgeon, 1992). A resolution of this problem is to acknowledge that there is, within grounded theory, a constant interplay between data and emerging theory which involves reflexive questioning as to how far there is 'fit'. Nevertheless, it is interesting to speculate how far I managed the 'fit': for example one of the variables I isolated was 'alliance between therapist and family members'. This concept is well known among family therapists and reflects the theoretical influence of Minuchin (1974). My 'discovery' does not imply that the variable is not 'real' or useful, simply that it is not original and was, perhaps, not derived solely through the grounded theory process.

Through being an insider, I addressed the point made by Bryman (1988) as to whether we can ever make interpretations that reflect the experience of those being researched. In Nagel's (1974) terms, can we ever say what it is like to be a bat? Nagel argues that we can to some extent roughly or partially try to take the bat's point of view, but then our conception will also be rough or partial.

As the therapist, I *was* the bat and could comment on the process of sessions from that perspective. I could bring my professional experience and judgement to bear and so inform the research through commenting on the process of the sessions.

QUALITY AND QUANTITY

Essentially, the quantitative part of the study was to identify the session outcome and the qualitative was to provide information as to why those outcomes occurred. The initial tension was between my understanding as to what would be considered credible research within the agency context and my need to understand what happened within the sessions through an interpretative method. In other words, I attempted to square the circle by opting for both quantitative and qualitative methods.

However, this led to a new tension, manifested as the problem discussed by Bryman (1988), of integrating quantitative and qualitative methods within a single study. Bryman argues that the epistemological positions underlying quantitative and qualitative approaches appear to be different paradigms. That is, within quantitative research a realist position is taken which assumes that there are facts out there in the world which can be discovered and represented as hard data. In contrast, a constructivist perspective often underlies qualitative methods. This approach focuses on how a situation is constructed by the active participants, and seeks to understand the social world via their accounts. However, researchers often run combined studies without recourse to this debate and so indulge in a technical integration. This is problematic if it is accepted that the method logically follows from the epistemological position; in other words, the methods must conflict as the epistemology does. However, Goodwin and Goodwin (1984) argue that the epistemology–method link is far from pure, and that methods may be used across the quantitative–qualitative divide. For example, grounded theory may be consistent with a constructivist position. Layder (1993) argues that Glaser and Strauss (1967) focus on grasping the meaning which emerges within the milieu investigated, rather than focusing on more objective measures. Conversely, it can be argued that grounded theory assumes that there are 'real' phenomena to be identified in the data from which theory can be generated.

Perhaps I was less able to live with the epistemology–method issues than Goodwin and Goodwin (1984), and this explains why I began to angle the qualitative data towards a quantitative paradigm. This showed in two main ways.

- Although there were qualitative assessments made by me of what was happening in the session, e.g. what constituted symptom-led communication, facilitated by my insider position, I developed a strong framework in the pilot study which was then used to analyse the sessions, i.e. there was a theoretical framework into which the process analysis could be fitted.
- I started to connect the themes of the session derived through the process study to the immediate session outcome, although this was a

qualitative approach, in addition to the directly quantitative single-case outcome measures.

Essentially, I was trying to increase the validity of the qualitative aspect by recourse to quantity, and in the process denying my position as an insider.

There are clear problems with reifying scientific objectivity. Science is itself a social process. What counts as good successful science is socially constructed and varies over time (Woolgar, 1993). This negates the use of quantity to validate qualitative work, as in my attempt described above.

It may be that I was simply too constrained at the outset to fully think through what a qualitative strategy would consist of. As well as agency constraints, my academic background is in psychology, which has not until recently adopted many qualitative methods. Perhaps I was subscribing to the myth that science somehow has a methodological superiority. The myth is maintained because the achieved moral order in natural science methods seems stronger and so able to resist deconstruction more easily (Woolgar, 1993).

The personal, agency and cultural contexts, the failure to adopt a new paradigm/grounded theory approach (Layder, 1993) and the use of a preconceived framework for analysing the data meant that the participants', i.e. the family's, understanding of the situation was never developed. There is an issue of researcher power that needs to be acknowledged here. The research merely replicated the current status quo of researcher dominance that Webb (1992) highlights. I maintained a distance from the family, even as a practitioner, in attempting to objectify the qualitative aspect of the study.

FORCED CHOICE

It is naive to think that research can ever take place in a political vacuum. Bryman (1988) recounts examples of where the appropriate method is chosen for the research question, but this may be a luxury to which research practitioners are denied access.

In the case of my research, by chance, the shift towards realism was less inappropriate as the therapy being evaluated and explored had itself realist underpinnings. (As the family therapist, I was using structural family therapy techniques which presuppose that there are certain observable, i.e. 'real' structures and relationships in all families, which the therapist seeks to modify in order to stop the presenting problem.) However, as I develop in practice my world view is shifting to a firmer, constructivist one, and in parallel my practice has become less directive. The distance between researcher and family in this research served to obscure important questions around the interaction of the participants in the therapy which my new perspective entails.

My role was crucial in helping to create the situation, and should have been a source of reflexivity and so greater understanding. In this circumstance there is an argument to be made for adopting a different research strategy. In particular an ethnographic approach would seem to offer the opportunity to understand the family's perceptions and interpretations of the therapy process. A strong ethnographic position denies that theory is either a goal, as in inductive social science, or a direction-giver to research, i.e. it rejects the hypothetico-deductive model of natural science. Description of a phenomenon is the means to increase understanding. Tesch (1990) uses an analogy to help justify the use of such qualitative methods: if one person had their portrait painted by many artists, each canvas would be an individual representation but it would nevertheless be recognizable as the same person.

WRITING THE CHAPTER

In the spirit of relexivity encouraged by this paper the last paragraph attempts a meta-analysis of the process of writing. To me, the following points seem cogent:

- It was easier to use the first person in the description of the qualitative work than in the quantitative, where I wanted to revert to the third person. I resisted impersonal pronouns most easily when presenting a critique of the quantitative model.
- It is clear that practitioner researchers can shift their world views as their academic/professional lives develop. This means that there will always be new interpretations placed on work undertaken. For example, this chapter differs from the written thesis and from the journal article based on the research. It is always possible to find better alternatives in retrospect.

CONCLUSION

From the outset there were clear agency expectations concerning what constitutes appropriate evaluation data, and I also carried a history of quantitative bias. This made the implementation of a qualitative approach difficult, despite my attempts at process study in an insider practitioner role which was to inform my practice. The tension was shown through by the way in which I tilted the data towards quantitative analysis. By chance this was consistent, because the grounded theory approach and conceptual framework used for data analysis was realist in orientation, and so in line with the single-case design. In other words, epistemological differences were minimized.

However, some of the benefits of gathering qualitative data were denied, i.e. in terms of richness and understanding. Thus, although there was insider expertise brought to bear in making sense of the process of the sessions, this was always qualified by the relation to either immediate or non-immediate session outcome measures, i.e. quantitative outcome measures. It seems that I vacillated along an insider–outsider continuum, but tended to settle overall at the outsider end.

As my world view has since shifted, it would be more consistent with the philosophical underpinnings of my family therapy practice to adopt a strong qualitative approach, e.g. an ethnographic approach and firm insider position, in order to increase the understanding of what happens within therapy, and to do this by drawing on the accounts of families and therapists and using these to inform the researcher's analysis. This would not result in prescriptions for how to do therapy, but would be presented as ideas to the community of practitioners to discuss and debate.

REFERENCES

Anonymous (1985) (with Sandra B. Coleman) We were somebody's failure, in *Failures in Family Therapy*, (ed S. B. Coleman), Guilford Press, New York, p. 278.

Beck, A.T., Ward, C.H.. Mendelson, M., Mock, J.E. and Erbaugh, J.K. (1961) An inventory for measuring depression. *Archives of General Psychiatry*, **4**, 561–71.

Bennun, I. (1986) Evaluating family therapy: a comparison of the Milan and problem solving approaches. *Journal of Family Therapy*, **8**, 243–52.

Birch, J. (1987) Waiting without purpose: a discourse on the Tao of Pooh. *Australian and New Zealand Journal of Family Therapy*, **8**, 143–8.

Bryman, A. (1988) *Quantity and Quality in Social Research*, Routledge, London.

Burnham, J. (1986) *Family Therapy*, Tavistock, London.

Elliot, R. (1983) Fitting process research to the practising psychotherapist. *Psychotherapy, Theory, Research and Practice*, **20**, 47–55.

Feyeraband, P.K. (1975) *Against Method*, Verso, London.

Friedlander, M.L. and Heatherington, L. (1989) Analyzing relational control in family therapy. *Journal of Counselling Psychology*, **36**, 139–48.

Frude, N. (1980) Methodological problems in the evaluation of family therapy. *Journal of Family Therapy*, **2**, 29–44.

Glaser, S. and Strauss, A.L. (1967) *The Discovery of Grounded Theory: Strategies for Qualitative Research*, Aldine Publishing Company, Chicago.

Goodwin, L.D. and Goodwin, W.L. (1984) Qualitative vs. quantitative research or qualitative and quantitative research? *Nursing Research*, **33**, 378–80.

Greenberg, L.S. (1984) Task analysis: the general approach, in *Patterns of Change*,(eds L.N. Rice and L.S. Greenberg), Guilford, New York, p. 138

Greenberg, L.S. (1986) Change process research. *Journal of Consulting and Clinical Psychology*, **54**(1), 4–9.

Gurman, A. and Kniskern, D. (1978) Deterioration in marital and family therapy: empirical, clinical and conceptual issues. *Family Process*, **17**, 3–20.

Heatherington, L. and Friedlander, M.L. (1990) Applying task analysis to structural family therapy. *Journal of Family Psychology*, **4**, 36–48.

Henwood, K.L. and Pidgeon, N.F. (1992) Qualitative research and psychological theorizing. *British Journal of Psychology*, **83**, 97–111.

Hersen, M. and Barlow, D.H. (1976) *Single Case Experimental Designs: Strategies for Studying Behaviourial Change*, Pergamon Press, Oxford.

Layder, D. (1993) *New Strategies in Social Research*, Polity Press, Cambridge.

Minuchin, S. (1974) *Families and Family Therapy*, Tavistock, London.

Nagel, T. (1974) What is it like to be a bat? *The Philosophical Review*, LXXXIII. Reprinted in *Readings in Philosophy of Psychology*, I, (ed N. Block), Harvard University Press, Cambridge MA.

Quinn Patton, M. (1988) *Creative Evaluation*, 2nd edn, Sage, London.

Parry, G., Shapiro, D. and Firth, J. (1986) The case of the anxious executive: a study from the research clinic. *British Journal of Medical Psychology*, **59**, 221–33.

Shapiro, M.B. (1961) A method for measuring psychological changes specific to the individual psychiatric patient. *British Journal of Medical Psychology*, **34**, 151–5.

Stevenson, C. (1993) Combining quantitative and qualitative methods in evaluating a course of family therapy. *Journal of Family Therapy*, **15**, 205–24.

Tesch, R. (1990) *Qualitative Research: Analysis types and Software Tools*, Falmer Press, New York.

Webb, C. (1992) The use of the first person in academic writing: objectivity, language and gatekeeping. *Journal of Advanced Nursing*, **17**, 747–52.

Woolgar, S. (1993) *Ethnography: a sceptical descriptive analysis of the taken for granted*, Unpublished conference paper, Qualitative Methods for Psychologists, Windsor, March 1993.

Introduction

We have put the following two chapters together because we feel that among the many ideas and issues that they raise, one strong connection between them is their discussion of practitioner values. Jean Davies was motivated to conduct her study because of the value that she places on promoting the health of women, and this is in turn linked to the ideological basis of midwifery as a profession – being 'with woman'. Ruth McKeown also held firm beliefs about practice, in her case about the way in which health promotion projects should be developed, namely that they should be client-led. Her practice values, however, were not necessarily the same as policy, and furthermore she was not sure whether they corresponded to the values implicit in research.

For both Ruth and Jean, however, their commitment to and involvement with their work put them in a unique position when it came to collecting data. As Jean describes, they were both in a position where they could carry out what we have called 'practitioner observation', in other words, they collected data as part of the research but also as part of their practice. In this way, their belief in and experience of client-centred practice substantially shaped their research strategies.

To those who adopt the notion of 'value-free science' this connection between values, methods and results seems somewhat disturbing. Ruth and Jean certainly seem like partisan researchers who have very firmly declared their position and their prejudices. However, at least they have declared their values openly, and we can read their work informed by our understanding of the positions they have taken. This is a luxury that is not often afforded to readers of research, who often have suspicions that the researcher has some particular axe to grind but can find no open discussion of this in the text. This openness therefore goes some way towards helping the reader to evaluate the research, by placing it in the ideological and practitioner context in which it inevitably exists. Values in research can have a strong effect on the way that data are collected and interpreted, and this is not always wholly positive – sometimes it is very easy to get carried away by crusading zeal. What we would argue here, using Ruth's and Jean's work as an example, is that values are not always 'contaminants' of research and can be worthy contributors, but that this is always easier to evaluate if they are made explicit.

CHAPTER 7

The health bus – a study of a developing project

Ruth McKeown

EDITORS' INTRODUCTION

When research is done by an outsider to an organization, it is well accepted that their presence has an effect on events within that organization. The presence of a stranger asking questions can often stimulate reflection and change in research subjects. When the researcher is an insider the position becomes even more complex. The researcher has an effect on events not only because they are a researcher, but also because they are a practitioner, and disentangling and identifying these effects can be extremely difficult. The problem is further compounded when, as in this study, the researcher is also a research subject; in other words, the researcher will collect data on themselves. Whereas the outsider negotiates access on their own terms and so can preserve the objectives of the research from the danger of 'going native', the practitioner researcher is already a native.

This scenario immediately raises concerns about bias and subjectivity. There is the undeniable issue of whether the data collected and, more importantly, the analysis and interpretation of those data, are due to what is 'really happening', or to the personal beliefs of the researcher. This observation may lead to recommendations that the research should avail itself of objective measures in order to 'control' bias, a recommendation that does not acknowledge that many objective measures are, in fact, subjective. In selecting measures in a research study there are always a number of choices to be made about the variables to be measured and the way in which this is to be done, choices which are ultimately dependent on researcher preference. Another proposed solution to control bias may be to bring in another researcher to collect or analyse data. This strategy may be possible if the project resources allow it, but it seems to run the risk of adding yet another set of observer effects to the study, which may be even more incalculable than those originally identified.

The qualitative solution proposed might be to exhort the researcher to concentrate on simple description, rather than interpretation – to let the data speak for themselves. It is, however, questionable as to whether data can ever do this and there are still choices about what to describe and how to describe it. Other strategies used to increase validity in qualititative research, such as 'immersion in the data', or 'developing intimate familiarity with the field' are nonsensical for a researcher who has been familiar with the field as a practitioner and who feels that, if anything, they are drowning in the data.

Controlling bias, therefore, seems to be a difficult task for any researcher and virtually impossible for the practitioner researcher. Furthermore, the ideal of bias-free research seems to conjure up a notion of a strangely distant researcher, viewing the world from the Olympian heights of objectivity and with no investment, or even interest, in the results of the study. This disinterested stance does not fit well with ideas about research as a means of improving or developing situations, although it may fit with ideas of research as being primarily to contribute to theoretical knowledge. If we accept practitioner research as arising from a concern or interest in the ways in which good practice can be developed, then it is clear that the practitioner researcher, even before the research begins, holds certain views or values about the nature of practice. As these values form the motivation for the research and the practice, we cannot expect that once the research starts they should be 'switched off'.

Practitioner values are a central issue in this study. The researcher was responsible for developing a particular health service which she tried to model in a way that supported her beliefs about what good health promotion should be about. The values that Ruth held, however, did not always fit in with policy and the nature of the project changed midway through the study because of management decisions. For the outsider doing research this would have been an interesting phenomenon to observe, but for Ruth this was an event which changed not only the research but also her practice.

It was possible, at this point, for the research to change direction to fit the new development, a strategy which would have produced a much tidier research report. What Ruth decided to do, however, was to continue her study of the process of establishing the service and to incorporate this change and her reactions to it into her account. The result was not only an account of the development of the service, but also an examination of the dilemmas faced by a practitioner who was required to work in a way that conflicted with her professional and personal values.

What emerges in this chapter is an examination of Ruth's beliefs and values which goes some way towards suggesting a solution to the problem of bias in practitioner research, which is not to see bias as simply a 'corrupting' influence on data, but as part of data. By examining the values she held, not only by introspection but by reference to the writing and ideas of others, Ruth effectively lays her cards on the table. This enables the reader not only to understand the process and motivation for the research, but also to put the research into perspective, allowing it to be evaluated within a particular context of values. This seems to be a more productive approach to the problem of bias, to openly analyse values rather than attempt to control or disguise them.

This type of analysis is difficult to do and is often uncomfortable for the researcher, yet it can avoid what is seen as the most serious problem of going/being native: 'identifying so much with the participants that, like a child learning to talk, he [sic] cannot remember how he found out or articulate the principles underlying what he is doing' (Silverman, 1985, p.105) Going native, in this description, is a problem because it can leave things unarticulated or unexplored which should be part of the research account. It is not the things themselves which are the problem, but the fact that they are not discussed or debated.

This clarifies the implications of practice values for practitioner research. Practice values are part of the world which is being studied and should be treated as such. In other words, they should be examined, discussed and evaluated as a fundamental part of the study, rather than ignored or disguised. This approach holds the possibility of two benefits. First, for the researcher it emphasizes an obligation to critically examine the assumptions that underpin the study, a process which leads to a more reflective piece of research. Secondly, this process of reflection allows the reader access to valuable data. The reader may not share the values of the researcher, but at least if they are articulated then the reader has some chance of evaluating them and taking them into account when evaluating the research as a whole.

INTRODUCTION

When I was first asked to contribute to this book I had initial doubts that my personal experiences in the field would be of any practical relevance. On further reflection, however, I considered that the validation of my experiences as a practitioner could be meaningful in the context of particular research problems. In this chapter I will consider some of the issues relating to my observations of the research process. I hope this will help readers to reflect on their own work and thereby reach a deeper understanding of the importance of examining the nature of their own involvement.

I am not attempting to be prescriptive in terms of methodologies or conclusions, since by its very nature this chapter is a personal view and does not reflect any firm belief system. As a manager within a district health authority health promotion service, in March 1989 I was asked to take charge of a new community-oriented project – a 'health bus', a mobile unit which would visit a range of communities. This presented me with the opportunity to develop a research project while a student in health and social research at the University of Northumbria. It is this research project and my relationship to it that is the subject of this chapter.

PROJECT HISTORY

When the project started it was a health project first and foremost, not a medical project, and its brief was to foster the health of people living in the most disadvantaged areas of the city of Sunderland. In this context health is understood as a positive state of wellness, something to be nurtured. The basic philosophy underpinning project work was to provide a multiagency approach to health promotion. A central feature was to be the partnership between the client (the community) and professionals, working together in imaginative ways to promote health. The project workers were to encourage client participation in all aspects of project life, including the evaluation process. The concepts of empowerment and autonomy were integral to work practice and this was set within a framework of community development.

In carrying out the study I was both researcher and project manager. In combining these two roles the intention was to spend one year studying the project in its embryonic form, evaluating activities and developments. This involved working directly on the bus with one other health promotion worker.

THE METHOD

The chosen method for the research was an ethnographic approach. Widely used in anthropological studies, this can provide detailed and reliable explanations for social or cultural events based on the beliefs and experiences of people within that culture. The ethnographer, who is concerned with observing behaviour directly in the natural setting, goes 'native' to experience and understand social meaning from the perspective of the inhabitants. Sustained and intensive observation is required in order to construct and interpret the data in context. The ethnographer engages in the process of reflexivity, by continually reflecting on situations, events, phrases, casual conversation and actions. This enables the appraisal of the reliability and validity of propositions made concerning behaviour. It also allows for a critical appraisal of methodological and other research issues.

The rationale for the use of this method in my research was primarily because the subject of study was a new and innovatory project which was being introduced into the community by a district health authority. The project, which was a health promotion mobile unit 'Health Matters', was initiated to test the viability of a bottom-up community development approach to health promotion. Embracing a participative style of working, the community-orientated strategy was intended to help local people articulate their own health priorities. This was to be achieved through a self-help process. It was therefore necessary to evaluate the impact of this project in terms of its value to the community in addressing the expressed health education needs of the local resident population. Examining the role of self help and professional involvement in this activity was a major aim of the study.

As manager of the project I thought I was in a good position to study, in depth, the underlying processes at work and provide what Geertz (1978) describes as 'thick description', which is essentially searching for the meaning underlying social action. The research was to be a longitudinal 1-year study, thereby providing ample time for this task. Also, achieving a naturalistic, interpretative account of the life of 'Health Matters' was a personal as well as a research goal. This was because, as a novice to social research, and ethnography in particular, I needed to extend my skills in this field.

Another reason for the ethnographic approach was that from my own experience I had observed that most of the studies within health promotion were predominantly quantitative in type. Although useful for measuring outcome or impact, questions are principally concerned with accountability, rather understanding how the programmes work. Process and important questions about quality are often ignored.

The innovative nature of the mobile project required that process be understood, and as manager I needed to be aware of its potential strengths and weaknesses in meeting particular goals. For example, it was important to know whether the non-traditional health care setting of the health bus influenced clients' perceptions of their role. Would the project encourage client self-empowerment to the point where they would be in a position not only to determine their needs but to find solutions to them? At the time, I believed that an ethnographic approach would be the most appropriate method for focusing on these areas.

GETTING STARTED

The first task was to look at relevant literature on the subject of health mobiles. In doing so it emerged that in Britain mobile work is not a new idea. In the late 1960s mobile services operated as part of government education priority programmes in urban areas. Since then mobile units have become more diverse and have been effective tools in different fields of work; mobiles have been used for play, library and art provision, through to crisis intervention services and health screening. The literature was thus helpful in illustrating the different types of mobile provision, highlighting their range and diversity, and it also indicated the potential benefits of mobile work to the client.

However, a problem I encountered in reviewing the literature was that very few of the studies on mobile work had given serious consideration to the role of the client. There was an implicit assumption, as in other forms of human service delivery, that the client (consumer) is a passive receiver. Service programmes were prescriptive in that they were planned and implemented by the providers, with little or no consultation with the client. There was little evidence, therefore, to support the idea that a mobile service based on community development principles would work. This gap in the research literature led me to question the validity of this approach for the project.

Despite the lack of supporting evidence, I held assumptions about the study which allayed these misgivings. First, I believed that health promotion practice which adopted a community-orientated strategy would be more effective in promoting health than health promotion that relied solely on top-down rationale-deductive strategic planning. Secondly, I believed that a mobile unit that took health promotion direct to clients, thereby putting professional resources at the clients' disposal, would be more successful in involving the clients in the evaluation process. Thirdly, I believed that information relayed by experts and passively received by participants confirms in the mind of the receiver that, in order to develop yourself, you have to be dependent on an expert. This then gives the expert the authority to determine the recipient's need. I therefore rejected the label 'consumer', on the grounds that the term depoliticizes individuals and removes responsibility for personal as well as communal health. Holding firmly to these beliefs, I had sufficient motivation to start what I viewed as a potentially challenging and exciting study.

METHODOLOGICAL ISSUES

A number of methodological issues emerged while I was engaged in carrying out the study. The first concerned my dual role as manager and researcher. As the ethnographer I was the methodological tool for constructing the data, and as manager of the project I was also a central character of the research. This led to inner confusion regarding the separation of these two roles. In the beginning the question would often arise, 'How do I do it?'. Even though I was a practitioner engaged in research I still held the perception of the researcher role as being separate and distinct from my position as manager. In my role as ethnographer, the participants would be regarded as objects of study, to ensure that my observations were also reliably objective. Effectively this also meant observing my own behaviour and interaction with others as manager. As manager, however, I was in a very subjective role. Immersed in daily activities and events, I was responsible for the development of the project and actively involved in directing the course of events, working to give clients some control over the project to create a service in which they had some ownership, rather than one that relied solely upon the expertise of the professionals involved. In other words, I was instrumental in changing the research setting, which resulted in my managerial position taking precedence over my role as researcher.

I also found that in trying to objectify my subjective managerial experience I was unable to capture the real meaning of this experience – the direct, intimate, experiential understanding in any theoretical formulation. It would somehow be diminished. When trying to resolve the role confusion I would experience inner tension and a sharpening of conflict, and for quite some time the two positions seemed irreconcilable. I eventually realized that my problem was one of conflicting views about this dual role, rather than actual confusion with the managerial and researcher roles themselves. With this realization I was able to relax and adopt the more flexible approach of the ethnographer.

The second methodological issue overlapped with the first and concerned the subjective nature of the research. In questioning my subjective position as manager, I experienced a sense of 'methodological distrust': questioning whether my construction and interpretation of the data provided an accurate account or whether it was simply a biased interpretation, influenced by my managerial position. In examining this problem I realized that the issue was first and foremost a philosophical one concerning the value of natural methods in social research. According to Bruyn (1970), this naturalistic model of enquiry is an 'inner perspective' methodology. From this position people are regarded as 'social beings with freedom and purpose as opposed to observing them deterministically as the product of external forces'. This view is further qualified by Denzin (1978), who suggests that the naturalistic interpretative approach 'reflects a respect for the phenomena of the everyday worlds of natural interaction'. One could argue that the subjective experience must then be one, if not the most, significant way to understand human behaviour.

I accepted implicitly the feminist concept of 'conscious partiality', the belief that the researcher is not separate from the research. At the very least the personal views of the researcher will be present, influencing the construction or interpretation of data. I also upheld the view that there is something to be found beyond the scope of what is being observed, unlike the positivist belief that there is nothing beyond the scope of the enquiry; that data are unchanged by the researcher's perceptions i.e. that observations can be objective without the intrusion of personal beliefs, values and presumptions. As more experienced researchers have shown, objectivity is an ambiguous concept, impossible to achieve in the social sciences because we cannot account for different interpretations of the same behaviour.

As the research evolved, however, I found myself holding less rigidly to my own preconceptions. I became aware of the project as a fluid, shifting process where nothing remained static or unchanged. It was something akin to what has been described as the 'simultaneity paradigm'. Simply, this means that people are in constant interchange with their environment in a process of synergy, moving towards meaning, connectedness and a commonality of direction and goal. If I held on to my assumptions and beliefs, therefore, I would observe the present process less clearly. By relinquishing preconceived ideas I found I became more open and aware of the actual process. By steeping myself in the events I could observe more fully the participants' involvement and draw from their experience a more naturalistic account. Yet as a completely inexperienced ethnographer with only textbook knowledge to draw upon, I was at the start unsure as to whether I had the necessary skills to put theory into practice.

What the experience taught me is that the ethnographer is consciously and subconsciously paying attention to all that is around, with intuition and cognition working simultaneously. This is nothing different from what we all engage in, but perhaps without the same degree of alert attention. In concentrating my efforts I began to notice an overall improvement in my observational and analytical skills.

Creative imagination was also stretched as spontaneous impressions of situations and intuitive insights arose, often not seeming to have any association with previous experience. Also, in trying to be sensitive to the situation and more empathetic towards others, this would contribute to a clearer understanding of what was happening and assist in bringing to light what was hidden. Essentially the ethnographer is trying to do what Becker and Geer (1972) describe as 'catching social reality in flight'. The goal is to discover what is happening and then to contextualize it by linking ideas or insights to known or emergent theoretical concepts.

The process of contexualizing ideas and insights, however, presented another methodological issue. In developing and refining ideas to fit them into what was already known about patterns of social action, I was in danger of distorting participants' meaning. So, in trying to provide high-level inferences and interpretations, I was never entirely sure that my interpretative account was validating the self-perceptions and experiences of the participants.

As time went by, I began to feel that the research agenda should have been internal to the group (participants). After all, the project goal was to 'foster professional–client collaboration and involve the latter in the evaluation process'. They ought then to have had a role in deciding the type of research to be carried out, which included the definition of purpose, the design and the discussion of implications and how policy could be influenced.

With the benefit of hindsight I now realize that an action (participatory) study would have been more appropriate. At the very least it would have allowed the subjective, socially constructed perceptions of participants to emerge without distortion. In addition, the study would have had more of a political character as participants assumed some responsibility for the direction and outcome of the study. As it was, a lack of insight concerning the participants' role in the research left the methodology unchanged.

Another methodological issue concerned the defining and operationalizing of concepts related to the main areas of project work. For example, the project brief was to support the development of self-help groups. As researcher I was to observe the developmental process of this activity, focusing on aspects such as group structure; how leadership emerges; how goals are set; group interaction, and so forth. A poor understanding of the varied definitions of self help, however, left me unprepared for the complexity of the self-help process that actually emerged. For not one but three types of self help were manifest in the project. First, there was self help of the kind that project workers were expected to promote, where people who had a common health interest met together to share experiences. Workers would support group activities from a peripheral position, to allow members adequate scope to assume their own roles within the group. It was the kind of activity that Reissman and Gartner (1987) refer to as 'helper therapy'.

A second type of self help emerged, however, exhibiting different features from the first. In this group members had a common health problem and, while providing mutual support, strong leadership emerged. They very soon acquired redefiner characteristics, viewing their health problem as being either created or exacerbated by external forces within the wider sociopolitical structure. They looked to project workers for advocacy rather than therapeutic support to ensure that their demands were channelled back to policy makers of statutory services. As I was an employee of the health service this created something of an ethical dilemma. To take on this advocacy or campaigning role could have been regarded as overtly political and threaten any future project funding. However, not to give support to members would have been to engage in discriminatory professional practice. As prior commitment had been given by workers to support their activities, there was no real decision to make. In the ensuing weeks, as membership grew, the group developed into a relatively autonomous entity, at which point members decided to move to a permanent static base. Project support was still given in terms of providing resources, while local community workers ensured that the advocacy role was maintained.

Although these two groups were being supported by the project, in general terms there seemed to be little self-help ethos in the poorer communities visited by the health bus. Clients who came on to the bus were mainly looking for satisfactory service delivery from health professionals. Most presented with a health problem or query, seeking alternative help. However, many of these clients would stay for long periods of time, talking to workers, and in doing so would often reach a clearer understanding of their problem. It was only in writing the final report that I realized that these clients had also engaged in a third form of self help, by actively seeking more information or explanations of their health problem or treatment. Unfortunately, I had failed to observe the actual process fully because of my initially poor grasp of the various definitions of self help.

DEVELOPING RESEARCH SKILLS

Throughout the duration of the study I never reached the stage of complete competence, and the development of my research skills was acquired slowly through intensive effort. To help me in the task I used different research techniques, which was useful for cross-checking the data and providing a monitoring device during the research process. To me this was important because, as the ethnographer, I was the main data-gathering instrument, which raises questions about accuracy, focus and observer bias, which are issues relevant to the study's reliability and validity. To counteract these problems I collected data from several sources, including informal interviews, participant observation, field notes and a diary. In this way I hoped to be able to triangulate data, by looking at the consistencies and differences between types of data.

The interviews presented no real problem and I have already indicated the difficulties concerning participant observation, in my role as manager. As for field notes, I found this to be an invaluable recording technique. Using the schema of Burgess (1988), daily notes were separated into three categories: description of the project, methodological issues and theoretical analysis. This format helped the reflexive process of continually reflecting on events, phrases, words used and conversation to get at people's meaning, which effectively helped to sharpen my observations. The methodological notes were especially useful for thinking about the validity of observations, while the theoretical notes helped to clarify meaning in a more structured and controlled way.

The main problem I encountered was with the diary: renowned as the valued tool of the ethnographer, I found it a burdensome chore, partly due to constraints of time, which I imagine is always a problem for the practitioner in research. Working full-time as manager, there never seemed enough time to jot items into the diary. I could manage the daily field notes, which I undertook at the end of the working day. The diary, however, was a different matter. As a means of recording events it had never appealed to me before and I regarded it as an activity that was only undertaken by people who enjoyed writing. The diary might be viewed by others as a creative and satisfying experience, but for me it was none of these things.

In saying this, however, I am not trying to decry the value or importance of this technique in research. It was very useful in that it did help to provide a historical account of events. It was also an aid to the reflexive process. However, given my disposition towards this recording technique, sustaining personal motivation was a constant problem. I persevered, but very inconsistently: sometimes a week or two would go by before an entry was made. On reflection, I realize that if my sole task had been to research the project, the experience could have been quite enjoyable. As it was, much of my energy was given to managing it, and trying to integrate this with what I considered was a rather time-consuming recording technique proved quite difficult.

In any event, after 6 months I had constructed a large amount of qualitative data elicited from various sources. In addition, a quantitative recording system was developed for collecting information relating to clients' usage of the project. While this data was being constructed and gathered, 6 months into the study the whole nature of the project changed.

THE IMPACT OF NEW POLICIES

As I indicated earlier, when the health bus started it had its own ideology which was akin to that of community development. Clients would be encouraged to develop their own programmes of health promotion with minimal intervention from health professionals. What the health bus was trying to do was to take health messages out of the health service and ground them in people's lives and environment. This is generally considered a good thing from a radical health promotion perspective, as it reveals a new way of thinking in health education, promoting positive interaction and communication between health professionals and local communities. This is a move which questions the individualistic approach and accepts the value of community action by those who experience social and other forms of disadvantage.

In a small way the project was beginning to make some progress in this direction, as self-help activity among some clients was slowly emerging, although in general terms, as I mentioned earlier, a self-help ethos was not particularly evident in the disadvantaged areas visited by the project. One of the problems was that, given the significance of social disadvantage and the impact of this on the clients' sense of wellbeing, the empowerment process was very hard to initiate. There was also the conflict between the policy-makers' perceptions of what the bus could achieve, clients' perceptions and bus workers' perceptions. The policy makers saw it as top-down delivery of services to a wide public, their needs having already been defined and packaged by managing professionals. The bus staff could see it as a potential for bottom-up policy, while the clients' preferences were not necessarily for the kind of self help that the researcher envisaged. In the end this conflict was to some extent resolved because of top-down policy change to a marketing structure.

With this policy change, areas of work were redefined and the focus for project work was now directed at reducing the high incidence of coronary heart disease in the Sunderland district. My own role as manager changed and I became responsible for devising, implementing and coordinating coronary heart disease prevention programmes. In this context the health bus became a resource for taking these pro-grammes out into the community. In practice this meant that the com-munity development principles upon which the project was based no longer existed. As researcher I faced a dilemma in not knowing how to proceed. I considered the idea of abandoning the study, as it seemed pointless to continue. How, for example, could I investigate the self-help process when it was no longer a feature of the project?

I also felt compromised by current changes, as I had worked hard to introduce into working practice a different approach to foster professio-nal–client collaboration and individual responsibility for health matters. Instead, the project was now implementing health promotion pro-grammes devised by professionals. The question was, would these programmes reflect the needs of the community or simply the expertise of the workers and traditional ways of working?

At this stage my concerns centred primarily on the project and its new direction, and the research became of secondary importance. Increasingly, I viewed the study as more of an academic exercise and this negative attitude lowered my motivation to continue with the research, so outside direction was sought. After some deliberation and consultation with my research supervisor, I decided to proceed with the study, first because I had already amassed a considerable amount of data, and secondly because there was still a process to be observed, albeit one that I had some misgivings about.

I decided against setting new research goals in favour of simply continuing the process of observing the events and activities of the project. As manager I was still fully involved in what I now rationalized as 'outreach' work. This new perspective was needed in order to replace the community development bottom-up approach and to sustain personal motivation.

It soon became apparent that the potential range of tasks was wide and included all kinds of activity, clinical medical interventions and non-clinical programmes of health promotion. The project now had a broad multipurpose character within which workers sought to link top-down with bottom-up approaches. Inevitably this was an uneasy alliance, because in the final analysis the efforts of the professional must fit in with the top-down policies which, to a great extent, are determined by macroeconomic factors. As far as the project workers were concerned, however, we had the resources and an understanding of community health issues. We were thus able to support community leaders, who had the trust and confidence of local people.

From the evaluation of the previous 6 months, I had recognized the value of working in close liaison and cooperation with community leaders. I had reached the conclusion that welfare professionals cannot simply open their doors and say 'What do you want?' or 'What are your health needs?' Before they can do this they have to stimulate interaction, possibly even suggesting issues that might hold latent concern; a two-way interaction is needed. Professionals need to have a rough idea of what issues concern people before any bottom-up strategy can be embarked upon. This is a lengthy process because it also involves the establishment of good working relationships and positive interaction with community leaders and the organizations they represent.

The task for the project was to now try and balance the rational deductive policy method with a bottom-up neighbourhood approach. This was helped in some way by the emergence of a new working premise from the evaluation – that project work could be carried out in the community through different organizations, utilizing major channels of the social structure, including educational, health and community services. In this way more people could be reached with newer, less traditional and more imaginative programmes of health promotion' e.g. puppet theatres for primary schools; a womens' health skills collective; assertiveness programmes for secondary school pupils; fitness testing for industrial employees; health road shows and music festivals. These programmes included a healthy lifestyle theme linked to coronary heart disease prevention. They were also integrated into a strategy which sought to encourage the development of public health policies, thereby addressing wider environmental and public health issues. This took the emphasis away from the 'victim-blaming' individualistic approach.

By consulting with community leaders and representatives from the various organizations, programmes of activity also reflected the interests if not the needs of the community. At the end of the first year I was relatively satisfied that the project was providing an accessible and flexible service to the people of Sunderland, proving its value in a number of respects. However, in relation to the study I was less convinced of its worth and considered it to some extent a failure, for the following reasons. First, as I indicated earlier, I was a completely inexperienced ethnographer. I viewed the research as a challenge but I lacked confidence in my research abilities, and because of this found it harder to be open and frank about the problems I was experiencing. My supervisor at the time was very supportive, providing me with useful and substantive ideas for improving the quality of my work, but I rarely expressed my real concerns. I learned mainly through trial and error, and my general lack of confidence in this area prevented me from seeking the required help. Invariably this underconfidence reflected in almost every aspect of the study, in the construction and interpretation of data as well as in the writing of the final report. Overall, my analysis of the project was simplistic and superficial.

Secondly, even though I attempted to address the methodological issues, there were areas of concern which I could not reconcile. For example, as the research progressed I felt very uncomfortable with the idea of 'doing research' on others. It seemed to contradict the idea of empowering clients, which was a principle the project tried to adhere to. As time went by I became more convinced that the process of empowerment is inhibited by treating participants as objects of study. The naturalistic research approach alleviated my concerns to some extent, but never completely, as sometimes my observations would be carried out in a covert manner.

Thirdly, as an evaluative study it lacked process measurements. Although I undertook low-level monitoring of the process, it would have been useful to set that against objective criteria or standards. Various conceptual models on evaluation exist, but none of these were integrated into the study, mainly because I was unaware of them at the time. A better understanding of what was involved in carrying out evaluation would have assisted the developmental and decision-making processes, ensuring that research participants had an active role to play in this regard. The introduction of such measures would have also shown whether the project was operating in its optimum form.

As it was I was the methodological tool for this ethnographic study and the data I had constructed offered very little protection against self-delusion. It was hard to know how much confidence to have in my own conclusions. By the end of the study I had amassed hundreds of notes which, in writing the final report, were reduced to a few uninspiring statements. The thought struck me that if I felt this way about the study, how much more so would the reader?

Had I been an experienced ethnographer, perhaps many of the problems I encountered would have been resolved much more quickly, but it is highly likely that such a background would have led to another set of problems. Instead of being too involved as a practitioner, I could well have been too distant as an ethnographer, and would not have had the professional experience and knowledge reqired to make some research decisions.

On reflection, if anything was achieved it was in the area of personal development. I can attribute to the ethnographic experience a heightened self-awareness; from the two-way interaction with participants, increased knowledge; and an overall improvement in research skills. I satisfy myself with the thought that in the final analysis, as a student in social research, this alone was sufficient justification for undertaking the study.

REFERENCES

Becker, H. and Geer, B. (1972) Participant observation and interviewing: a comparison, in *Symbolic Interaction,*(ed B.M. Meltzer), Allyn and Bacon.

Bruyn, S.T. (1970) The new empiricists: the participant observer and phenomenologist, in *Qualitative Methodology,* (ed W.J. Filstead), Markham Publishing.

Burgess, R. (1988) *Studies in Qualitative Methodology,* Jai Press, Greenwich, Conn.

Denzin, N.H. (1978) *Sociological Methods,* 2nd edn, McGraw Hill, New York.

Geertz, (1977) *Interpretation of Cultures,* Basic Books, New York.

Riessman, F. and Gartner, A. (1987) The Surgeon General and the self help ethos. *Social Policy,* **18,** 23–5.

Silverman, D. (1985) *Qualitative Methodology and Sociology: Describing the Social World,* Gower, Aldershot.

CHAPTER 8

A study of family networks and relationships in community midwifery

Jean Davies

EDITORS' INTRODUCTION

In this chapter Jean Davies describes a study that she undertook in order to explore family networks in the community in which she worked. Her interest in this aspect of the neighbourhood arose from the conversations and experiences that she had had visiting women and their babies over a period of 4 years as a midwife. In Jean's study practice was clearly a stimulus for research but, as her chapter shows, the relationship between research and practice was more complex and intimate than this. Jean uses the phrase 'practitioner observation' to describe this relationship, and this exemplifies some of the issues at the heart of practitioner research. Many readers will be familiar with the term 'participant observation', which is used to describe a method of collecting data in qualitative research. In participant observation the researcher enters a field as a participant; in other words, they take part in the activities that they observe. This may vary from complete participation, where the researcher acts as a full member of staff, for example, or there may be some limits imposed on the participation that occurs, and the researcher may restrict their activities to well-defined areas. Whatever the role chosen, the principles of participant observation are that the researcher is immersed in the world that they are studying, in order to gain an intimate familiarity with it and to collect detailed data. The data that are collected in participant observation are not just confined to records of behaviour – the researcher can also access and collect other types of data, ranging from informal interviews and conversations to documentary data, organizational policies and official statistics, as they present themselves during the course of the study. Participant observation, therefore, can be a rich source of naturally occurring data.

Participant observation, however, is directed and determined by the aims of the research. In practitioner observation, the researcher is present primarily as a practitioner rather than as a researcher, and it is the practitioner role that takes precedence. Information collecting, therefore, is determined not by research interests but by the interests of practice. Practitioners are granted access to a variety of types of information, and indeed have a responsibility to acquire information, but this is because of their practitioner role rather than any research role. Practitioner observation therefore accesses a great deal of data, but it is not precisely focused on research aims. Whereas it is possible to be selective in the collection of data in participant observation, selectivity in practitioner observation is often restricted to the data analysis stage. In other words, the vast amount of data that practitioner observation accrues is often only tangentially related to the focus of the research, and this requires practitioner observers to sift through the data in order to illuminate their research. In many ways, as Jean points out, it may be useful to think of such data as being secondary, collected for purposes other than research.

Practitioner observation depends on attentive practice (see also Chapter 9), which incorporates the skills of listening, observation and paying attention to and questioning what is going on. These skills are, of course, what we would hope for anyway in a practitioner, a point which again illustrates the link between research and practice – it does not seem likely that someone who has not developed these skills in practice will suddenly display them when doing research.

When discussing practitioner observation Jean also highlights the importance of professional values in both practice and research. She is very clear about the philosophical underpinning of midwifery – that it is to be 'with woman' – and extends these values to practitioner research. If the purpose of midwifery is to be with women, then the purpose of midwifery research is to help midwives to be with women. This discussion of values as a guide to developing and evaluating research is very different from ideas that we have described elsewhere about research as 'value-free' (see Chapter 3 for further discussion). The traditional response to Jean's discussion would be, of course, to argue that values have no place in science and that they constitute a source of bias which must be controlled as far as possible.

As Jean's chapter shows, however, practitioner research is not necessarily a way of perpetuating professional biases. It does not simply reinforce prejudices and assumptions, because the researcher cannot see beyond immediate practice mores. Indeed, as Jean describes, her data challenged many of her assumptions. She talks about the impact of particularly dramatic cases – she gives the example of the woman with nine children by three different fathers – which can colour practitioners' ideas of their clients. As her research shows, however, these stereotypes can be challenged by an examination of the more mundane cases: in her research she found that 73.8% of the siblings in her study had the same father and that 70% of the women had a stable relationship.

This process of using research to confirm and challenge observations made in the course of practice mirrors to some extent the discussion in Chapter 3 about small-circuit and long-circuit reflexivity. Initial impressions perhaps correspond to small-circuit reflexes, in which fast decisions are made that they help practitioners to function in their work. Long-circuit reflexivity, however, is more contemplative and research can be used as an aid to this contemplation, in which impressions are examined more closely. This perhaps gives us an indication of the criteria that we might use to evaluate practitioner research, that there is evidence that conclusions have been arrived at by a process of challenging ideas rather than accepting them as 'self-evident'.

Another interesting idea that Jean discusses is the contrast between holistic and reductionist modes of research. Instead of following a biological sciences mode of research, in which attention is paid only to a narrowly defined area of study, Jean advocates a much wider approach as being more appropriate for health care research. In her study she extended the notion of holism not only to the study of whole individuals, but to a study of the way in which they lived in family and community networks. This extended notion of holism offers opportunities for practitioner research to address wider social and political issues, by extending studies into these areas. Although much practitioner research is, understandably and appropriately, confined to small samples in specific settings, it does not always follow that wider issues cannot inform and be informed by the research.

Jean has not done a national survey of family networks or the relationship between patterns of house occupancy and poverty, but her research still has something to say about these issues. As we have mentioned elsewhere (for example in Chapter 11), the use of illuminative studies to inform practice in other settings does not rest on traditional notions of generalization and random sampling. Midwives working elsewhere will find the study useful in that it encourages them to think about their clients, rather than because the results are statistically significant and so, in orthodox thinking, can be 'generalized' to a wider population.

INTRODUCTION

This study was stimulated by observations that I had made in my practice as a midwife on a housing estate in Newcastle. Many of the women that I visited seemed to be related to each other, and the impression I had was that I worked in area with a resident population which was closely related and relatively stable – people did not seem to move from the area, although they did appear to move house within it. This seemed to be such a distinctive feature of the community that I decided to follow up my impressions by a more systematic study. I felt that I needed to clarify my impressions in order to learn more about the women that I worked with. As a midwife my primary interest is with the health of women and their children, but in order to promote health it seemed to me that I needed to develop a clearer understanding of the social and familial circumstances in which they lived.

Modern views of the family often portray it as a disintegrating struc- ture – the picture is often painted of families separated by great dis- tances, with members unable or unwilling to communicate with or support each other. As a consequence health care initiatives tend to look at clients on an individual basis, and staff assume that they will be the primary source of support and help. This, in many ways, fits in with reductionist medical models of health, in which intervention is not only aimed at individual people, but often at individual organs. As a commu- nity midwife, however, I am committed to holistic approaches to health care and I extend this holism not only to whole individuals, but to the communities and networks in which they participate. If my impressions of a closely related community were supported, then this would enable me not only to adapt my practice accordingly, but also affect how health care services in this area developed.

THE RESEARCH SETTING

I was working and continue to work as a community midwife in the area of the city where I did this research. From 1983 to 1987 I was one of four midwives employed with the Newcastle Community Midwifery Care Project. This project was to assess the impact of giving enhanced midwi- fery care to women identified from the 1981 census as having above average rates of social and economic deprivation (Evans, 1987). The research described in this chapter was undertaken following the com- pletion of this project; the interest in the networks and activities grew as a result of working with it.

I worked in one area, Cowgate, which is a clearly defined location, bound on three sides by roads and on the fourth by the Town Moor. This is a piece of land secured for pasture belonging to the Freemen of the City from medieval times, on which cattle graze, hence the name Cowgate. The estate was built in the 1930s and is laid out in the garden suburb manner, with most houses having gardens. It has an open aspect over the Moor and should be a desirable place to live. However, unem- ployment and many of its associated problems had a detrimental effect on the area and it began to have an identity of its own, which became reinforced by stigma, and it became known as not a good place to live.

The figures in Table 8.1 were provided by the Housing Department of Newcastle City Council and illustrate the economic standing of the estate in comparison with the city council tenants as a whole.

Table 8.1 Comparison between Cowgate and other Newcastle estates, 1989

	Cowgate	*City*
	%	%
Unemployment		
% of potential workers	85.5	21
Tenants on housing benefit	99	64
Current rent arrears	65	45
(Average arrears	£285	£154)
Tenants > 5 years	95	39

Newcastle City Council 1989

There is currently a massive upgrading of the area, with a huge injection of government money. However, the research in this chapter preceded this development. It is the intention to repeat the work when the work is complete to see what changes have occurred as a result.

THE STUDY

During the 4 years of the project it became obvious that the family networks were a crucial factor in the lives of the women in Cowgate, and I decided to study them in order to understand more about how this particular social group functioned. With another midwife, I was responsible for all the women in the area who were having babies. We visited them all at home during their pregnancy and after they returned home from hospital with the baby. I was also instrumental in establishing a Neighbourhood Centre with the local Social Services Department, with whom there was a shared philosophy of promoting health through raising self-esteem.

Anthropology might seem to be the discipline which has the most to offer in the way of theoretical support for the task of looking at kinship networks. However, it was not just the networks that were of interest but also how they related to activities and the perception of health. An anthropologist would study a community through the ethnographic collection of detailed data about its members; a sociologist would study interaction between them and a psychologist would try to understand how they function, both individually and within the groups. A midwife, however, has a primary interest in the way that women function within their family during childbirth and pregnancy, and it was this professional perspective that provided the impetus for this study.

Having worked in the area for 4 years I already had a lot of information, but it had not been collected systematically and was often at the level of verbal networking: of knowing that so and so was related to that son of so and so whose mother and aunt lived in such and such a place. The knowledge gathered was also not just about the kinship networks, but was specifically about a childbearing group of women. The research was essentially midwifery research, taking its definition from the official UKCC statement on the role of the midwife, that along with the specific tasks relating to pregnancy, birth and the postpartum period, 'She has an important task in health counselling and education, not only for the patients, but also within the family and the community' (UKCC, 1991).

Midwives are in a unique position and work with individuals and families at a time of heightened emotional sensitivity, and have a particular role in the dynamics of the family. Most professions are more 'other' than the midwife, whose fundamental remit is to be 'with' woman. This enables a particular kind of observation and experiential learning. Accumulating knowledge through practice is not abusing a privileged position, it is the professional necessity of the practitioner. It is also imperative for every profession to have research based on their particular practice and, as far as midwifery goes, this means understanding the cultural dimension of the families with whom the midwife works. One way of gathering such information and formulating it into a theoretical framework is through practitioner observation.

METHODOLOGY

The research looked into the family networks and activities of 80 child-bearing women, taken from a possible cohort of 180 who had delivered a child or children between 1983 and 1988. They all lived in Cowgate council estate and had all been cared for by me in my capacity as community midwife during their pregnancy and postnatal period. The estate consisted of 1000 properties, all but nine being council-owned. Only one woman in the study was not a council tenant. Ninety percent had lived on the estate for more than 5 years and 45% had been there for more than 16 years, probably all their lives. Seventy-six of the 180 identified women had moved off the estate and were excluded from the study; 23 were not interviewed because of time constraints, and one was abandoned after several attempts, as she was either 'just on the way out' or 'had just come in'. This left 80 women who were studied. Written consent was given by all women following an explanation about the study. There were no refusals, though one woman said she did not want me to come back to tell her she was 'related to every Tom, Dick and Harry on the estate'.

The study consisted of three parts, a questionnaire, a mapping exercise, and observation.

Questionnaire

A questionnaire was developed from which data about family networks and activities were gathered, about family connections within the estate and the frequency of contact. There were also some open- ended questions about health perceptions, problems and behaviours. There were questions about diet, smoking and exercise. Finally there were questions about housing activities on the estate, i.e. the patterns of house occupancy and house moving.

Table 8.2 shows the amount of contact with parents, as frequent contact, particularly with mothers, was common. Table 8.1, comparing Cowgate with other tenants, also shows that there was less movement than in other areas of the city.

Table 8.2 Parents on the estate and frequency of contact

	Mother %	Father %
Living on Estate	43.8	31.8
Daily contact	53.8	33.8
Weekly contact	26.3	12.5
Monthly	5	
No contact	6.3	23.8
Parent dead	8.8	26.3
In prison		1.3

What surprised me was the number of parents who had died, given that 95% of the women were under 35. This is perhaps a localized example of the effect of poverty on longevity, as the parents were reported to have died in their 50s and 60s.

When looking at the marital status of the women, 65% were not married. However, only 27.5% could be said to be living alone. This figure included 17.5 who lived alone, 8.8 divorced and 1.3 widowed, and 2.5 whose partners were in prison, which meant that over 70% were in fact living in a some form of stable union.

However, the impact of family on the perception of wellbeing was significant: 60 women indicated in the questionnaire that they experienced problems in their lives, and their descriptions of their primary or main identified problems were coded into the categories shown in Table 8.3.

This table shows that family and partners together form the largest group of problems mentioned by the women in the questionnaire (25), but an examination of some of the problems classified into other groups indicates that they were also linked to family issues. Housing problems, for example, arose for some women because of changes in family structure, such as relationships breaking up. Financial problems too could be family related, in that they could arise from the costs of providing for children, or from the inability to find a job to support the family.

Health problems were identified by the women themselves and also from their responses to other items in the questionnaire. Some of the questions about lifestyle indicated that there were health problems as health professionals usually define them: of the 80 women studied only 19 did not smoke, that is, 76% of them did; 52.5% had eaten no fruit or vegetables the day before completing the questionnaire and 90% had had no exercise the week before completing the questionnaire. There was also evidence of a high use of health services: 58.8% had either seen their GP in the surgery or had called them out in the week prior to the interview; 40% had visited the hospital in the week of interview: seven women were visiting others, and others attended for ongoing treatment; one woman had been in hospital for a tubal ligation but had fled because the woman in the next bed had frightened her. This large number using the NHS raises the question as to how effective this contact is, particularly when the 'health' problems mentioned by the women are generally outside the remit of medical practitioners.

Among the problems identified by the women as health issues were the following: three women were suffering from domestic violence; two were having a sexual relationship with the same man, who was in trouble with the police on drug-related charges; two women had partners in prison; one woman's stepchild was being encouraged to steal by a partner who was subsequently imprisoned for child abuse; and unemployment was causing depression in one family who had previously had a good work record. In addition; two women had children involved in child abuse cases, one where the abuser was an ex-husband and one where it was a neighbour, and the police were involved. One woman had been abused as a child; two were simply finding the family 'too much'; one woman was concerned about a sister who had had a stillborn child and whose boyfriend was on drugs; two women were disturbed by family rows about girls in the family becoming pregnant; two women reported that their children were disturbed; and one woman's child had died from leukaemia.

As can be seen from this catalogue of disasters, there is very little

Table 8.3 Types of primary identified problems

	Family	Partner	Finance	Health	Housing	School
N = 60	11	14	9	20	5	1

within these dis-ease-making situations that lies within the remit of the prescribing general practitioner. The women in the study classified these problems as health problems, yet they do not match with the services provided by health practitioners – indeed, it is difficult to think of a service that could meet these needs. What does emerge, however, is that the women use a broad definition of health and include many psychological and social problems under this umbrella term. In this sense they may be using a more holistic model than health care practitioners, but they have little power to have their ideas recognized or used to shape health services.

Mapping

Maps were constructed to represent the family networks and housing activity graphically. A stylized map was drawn of the estate, showing each dwelling. The original plan as far as the mapping went was to start with one family, interview them, and from this information map out the homes of their family connections. These relatives would then be visited and the homes of their family connections would be mapped, and the process would continue until the family network was exhausted. This method became too complicated and messy: Figure 8.1 illustrates the extent of the web of connections within the estate that was not continued because it became like the proverbial kitten in a ball of wool. This map resulted from three rounds of data collection, i.e. it started off with one couple in their home, mapped their relatives and then their relatives' relatives, illustrating the density and complexity of family networks in Cowgate. Even when the actual geography of the area (as represented in an Ordnance Survey map, for exmple) was modified in order to present a stylized map, it is still difficult to read.

The mapping method subsequently adopted was a more restricted placing of specific family relationships on a map of the area. First, as a general indicator of the number of immediate family connections, 10 randomly chosen women's immediate family networks were looked at together, and there were 104 households (out of the possible l000 on the estate) that were connected. The pervasiveness of family connections was highlighted when a subsequent 10 women's networks were examined, only three of whom were not interconnected with the previous 10. Specific relationships, namely mother/daughter and sister/ sister relationships were mapped out for those women in the study who

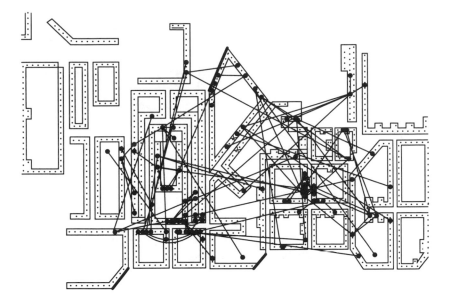

Fig. 8.1 First attempt at mapping.

had these relatives living in Cowgate (see Figures 8.1 and 8.3, in which the stylized Cowgate map has been omitted in the interests of clarity). It was not possible to incorporate into the mapping any indication of the closeness of these contacts – some may have been very intimate and others may have involved only infrequent contact, but this type of data would have been extremely complicated to collect, interpret and present. What emerged, however, was that the women in the study did have a large number of relatives living in the Cowgate estate. The total number of sisters identified in the study was 84, distributed over 81 houses, and the mother/daughter maps revealed that there were 27 mothers identified in the study and 37 adult daughters.

Observation

Working clinically with a group makes participant observation of a particular order (in the discussion later I develop the 'practitioner observation' concept), as interaction is largely determined by clinical imperatives. This can lead to the accumulation of a vast amount of data, but this collection cannot be as research-focused as it is when the researcher is only present for research reasons. The data collected in what I have called practitioner observation is in many ways similar to the definition that Glaser (1963) gives of secondary data, that is, 'Existing data which were originally collected for other purposes', which gives rise to all of the problems of selection and analysis that Reed (1992) describes.

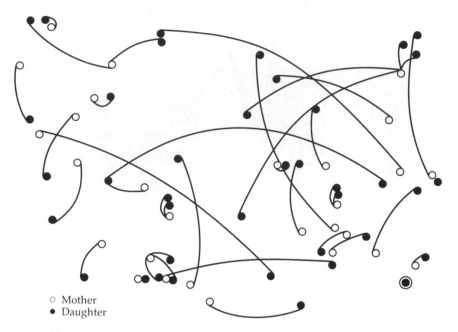

○ Mother
● Daughter

Fig. 8.2 Mothers and adult daughters living in Cowgate.

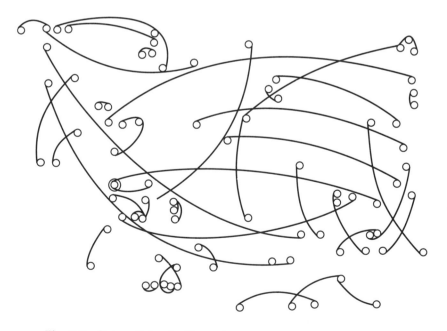

Fig. 8.3 Sisters living in Cowgate.

Practitioner observation, then, is similar to traditional participant observation, in that it draws upon many different types of data, observation of activities, conversations with participants, information about the setting and documentary data (see, for example, Denzin, 1978). However, the focus in participant observation is the research aim, however loosely this is defined, whereas in practitioner observation the reason for seeking information is to facilitate practice. This means that the practitioner researcher must subdue research interests in order to prioritize practice, and is often left with a mass of data which is completely unshaped to the research.

For example, one of the observations that was made in the course of practitioner observation was that people moved house very frequently, as was evident from client records and the midwives' diary entries of unsuccessful visits to clients' old homes. The information that I had, however, had been collected in an ad hoc way and was not easily adapted to the research study. I therefore developed some of the questionnaire items to flesh out this information and to gain a more systematic picture of house moves. The interplay between data collected from practitioner observation and more explicitly research-oriented activities can be illustrated by the example of one woman who, when visited, could not remember where she had moved from. As I had visited her in her previous house, I was able to fill in the gap for her by looking at my records.

The frequency of house-moving within the estate appeared to be a particular feature of how the women coped with living on the estate. These maps illustrate the number of house moves the women had made in the previous 5 years. Figure 8.4 illustrates one group of 16 women's house moves.

They follow a similar pattern and create an impression of people 'skittering' about. Despite this constant apparent movement, there was a feeling of no-one going anywhere and the frequency of contact with parents is an indication that there was very limited social mobility. Developing this idea more theoretically, it is possible that this house changing might perhaps have been some form of response to their situation – it may have helped against being dragged down by the palpable debt and poverty many were experiencing. This skittering about on the surface may have stopped them sinking into a sense of hopelessness.

The house-moves map therefore helped to formulate a tentative theoretical framework for thinking about about how the women survived the long-term hopelessness of their poverty, and it helped me to think about other aspects of my practice. For example, I had been puzzled as to why parentcraft classes were so different from others that I had taught over the previous 10 years. Topics would be tossed aside and it was difficult to maintain any theme as the women moved on to more immediate

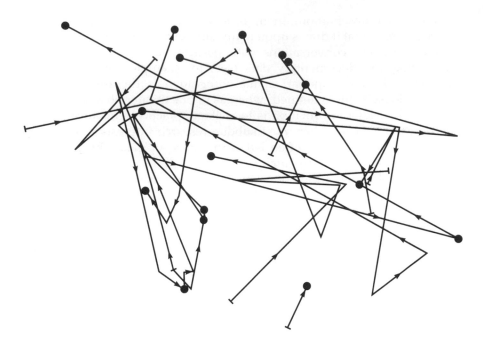

Fig. 8.4   House-moves map.

topics, such as what had happened on the previous night out on the street. The house-moving maps looked as if they displayed a similar pattern of activity, moving frequently for a 'new start' but with no real change from the old: very similar to the discussions in parentcraft classes, which flitted from topic to topic but did not really change people's ideas or give them new knowledge.

This 'going nowhere' is also perhaps reflected in the way in which the women used health services, with women going to the GP but having problems which were often out of the range of the possible strategies available. The women would go to the GP but their visits would not make any difference to their health – their problems were largely social ones. Again, there was a lot of surface activity in going to the surgery, but little real change.

PRACTITIONER OBSERVATION

Practitioner observation is a means of gathering data which is different from participant observation in that the practitioner has a clear role in the provision of health care. This means that the practitioner observer is privy to information because of their practitioner role, rather than because of their research role. Practitioner observation therefore has a different dimension to it, in that the relationship is particular to the work in hand.

Midwifery is the oldest health profession. There is no ambivalence about the role: people know what a midwife is and working in a neighbourhood meant that there was easy access to information. Consequently a lot of knowledge about the families was accumulated, not just on an individual basis but also about the neighbourhood. The family networks that were evident were interesting not only in their closeness but in the extent to which they were pervasive throughout the estate. The comment by a housing official that if a particular family continued to reproduce at the present rate they would soon have a member in every house on the estate set the scene for trying to discover how true this comment might prove to be.

Gathering data from clinical contacts raises the ethical issue about information given and received at the professional interface. Clients give such information to practitioners on the understanding that it is to be used for clinical purposes, and so they cannot be presumed to have consented to this information being used for research. In practitioner research, however, the boundaries between research and practice become blurred, as the purpose of such research is to inform practice.

The information that clients give for clinical purposes increases the body of knowledge in that particular field of practice, and much research is based upon or stimulated by clinical experience. The medical clinician, for example, learns experientially about whatever specialism he or she is involved in. This, in turn, becomes recognized through exposition of the work, which is developed through research and theories will be tested and subjected to trial and error; perhaps all science is experiential in the first instance. Clinical problems are the forerunners of controlled trials.

Experiential knowledge, gained through working with people in their own environments, is beginning to be given the same credence as work done in the isolation of the 'pure' scientific laboratory. This is no more necessary than in matters relating to health; the time should have passed when the social context was ignored as being central to the wellbeing or otherwise of a person.

Each day midwives learn from mothers, babies and families, and this is done on an individual basis. However, mothers and families belong to communities, and to learn about them it is necessary to study them in a systematic way. Without this it is possible that the more colourful occurrences and families assume a position that is out proportion, and stereotypes can grow, often creating a completely false image as a result of prejudice and the lack of understanding of cultural phenomena.

CONCLUSION

Nursing and midwifery are becoming more confident about their knowledge and are building a research base. They both have a long history of practice-derived knowledge, much of which has not been subjected to research, but it has worth that is waiting to be proven in an orthodox scientific way. There is a need for the foundations and theoretical structures of practice to be acknowledged and developed, a process which can be both exciting and painful. Some practices may be discarded in the light of research, but research will also be an affirmation of good practice.

Midwifery has a traditional position in society: the wise woman of the neighbourhood who dealt with birth and who also often laid out the dead was sometimes held in awe, not least because she knew so much about the people with whom she worked. There is more social fragmentation today, but the midwife is still part of the social structure. She can see the family function in its most fundamental way. Visiting a new mother whose partner you have also seen in exactly the same role with another woman tells you something about that family. If this occurs more than once in a small community with several fathers it may begin to tell you something about the community, not least that there are some complicated networks in the making.

Most midwives have been privy at some point to confidences a mother will share with no-one else. However, in order to establish whether this is a common situation, rather than letting an impression grow into a prejudice which might be coloured by personal opinion, it would seem to be a requisite for a community midwife to establish what are the cultural mores of those among whom she works. In this research, for example, only 35% of the women were married but 70% were in stable unions. The average number of children for the group of women was 2.9; 73.8% of these sibling groups had one father. Drama dictates that it is the woman with nine children with three fathers that is easy to recall, but the data from the other women shows above all else that she is not typical. In this way research can develop ideas and impressions into a more systematic understanding, which might be less interesting but is far fairer on the group, who are stigmatized already by their economic situation.

The research also highlighted the fact that, despite having worked with all the women already, a lot of information was not known, even though there had been professional contact. Family connections that existed simply had not been noted because of different names, or because families had fallen out. To have a clearer picture of the cultural background of women's lives a systematic approach must be taken. You cannot really be 'with' women if there is a lack of understanding about their lives, be it within an ethnic minority or a subcultural group within an indigenous population. This study did not therefore simply confirm my original impressions, but it added to my stock of knowledge about the community in which I worked.

Gathering information from among people that you have already worked with is very satisfying, as you have the opportunity of confirming what you only had an inkling about: that Barbara X and Shelly Y are cousins, and their mother is married to the brother of Bobby Z who is the father of . . . and so it goes. . . . And did you know that? . . . and who said what to whom. In an area where the economic framework is so fragile and mobility very limited these kinships become the very structure of the community. Through the systematic drawing of the networks for 80 women it was possible to form a wider and more accurate picture of the social makeup of the estate, being aware that at the end of the day this is a description not a definition of the people there. The value of this type of knowledge for a midwife is considerable, given that a midwife needs to be aware of the social environment if she is to know the pregnant women in her care.

Health has a cultural base and in order to begin to understand how it is perceived and, therefore, where and whether it might be possible to introduce new concepts, it is essential to address this cultural dimension. This work was not an anthropological study but a study developed from midwifery, using some anthropological and sociological techniques but developing theories to progress professional practice. Medicine reinforces and develops its knowledge base through the scientific route, which is well trodden and has its self-supporting structures. Its research often 'follows' clinical practice and it is one of the necessary steps up the career ladder which helps the individual researcher enhance their professional standing.

Medical research tends to be reductionist, following the scientific foundations of the biological and physical disciplines upon which it is based. Midwifery and nursing research, however, is unlikely to be reductionist, as they are founded in the humanities and their research needs to develop its own methodologies, reflecting the particular social interactions which are their dynamic. There are, of course, clinical procedures that can and should be subject to rigorous testing, which will affect the way that care is given. It is also true to say that research into midwifery and nursing must be systematic and consistent, but nursing and midwifery research must develop its own criteria, not based on a medical model, which should be as rigorous but different.

The difference is that philosophies can be illustrated by two quotations, both about teaching, by which the precepts of a profession are passed on. The first is from the Hippocratic Oath, which is still thought of as being the foundation of medical ethics.

To impart to my sons and the sons of the master who taught me and the disciples who have enrolled themselves and have agreed to the rules of the profession, but to these alone, the precepts and the instruction

(Darton, Longman and Todd, 1981)

The second quotation is from the *Medieval Woman's Guide to Health*

I therefore shall write somewhat to cure their illnesses, praying to merciful God to send me grace to write truly to His satisfaction and to the assistance of all women. For charity calls for this; that everyone should work to help his brothers and sisters . . . and so, to assist women, I intend to write of how to help their secret maladies so that one woman may aid another in her illness and not divulge her secrets to such discourteous men . . . who love women only for physical pleasure and for evil gratification . . . and fail to realise how much sickness women have before they bring them into this world.

(Rowland, 1981)

This difference in approach continues to this day and is reflected in how some research develops. The research discussed in this chapter showed that health issues cannot always be seen in purely medical terms. It also showed that the cultural identity of a group of people is not immediately obvious to those working with them: the professional view may be a response to the drama of the different, but on reflection the differences may be observed without prejudice.

With thanks to Dr Brian Bell of the University of Northumbria, for his supervision and support.

REFERENCES

Darton, Longman and Todd (1981) *Dictionary of Medical Ethics*.
Denzin, N. K. *Sociological Methods*, 2nd edn, McGraw-Hill, New York.
Evans, F. (1987) *An Evaluation Report. The Newcastle Community Midwifery Care Project*, Newcastle Health Authority, Newcastle.
Glaser, B. G. (1963) Retreading research materials: the use of secondary analysis by the independent researcher. *American Behavioral Scientist*, **6**, 11–14.
Reed,J.(1992) Secondary data analysis in nursing research. *Journal of Advanced Nursing*, 17(7), 877–83.
Rowland, B. (1981) *A Medieval Woman's Guide to Health*. Croom Helm, London.
UKCC (1991) *Midwives' Code Of Practice*, United Kingdom Central Council for Nursing, Midwifery, and Health Visiting, London.

Introduction

One of the potential dangers of practitioner research is that it can become too complacent. Practitioners can become so convinced that they are acting in the best interests of the client that they can often forget to confirm that their assumptions or views coincide with those of the client. It is therefore quite possible that practitioner researchers can fail to listen to clients and, even worse, fail to realize that they have made this omission.

Both the chapters in this part are about listening to clients. In Debbie Skeil's research the assumption that people with similar health problems will like to be together – an assumption that has gained ground over the years as self-help groups have grown – is challenged by her findings, which indicate that this is not always the case. In Sarah Huckle and Bob Heyman's study the data suggest that many of the ways in which professionals care for people with learning difficulties are not greeted with enthusiasm or approval by these people or their informal carers. In both studies the aim has been to examine critically some of the assumptions that underpin practice.

Challenging long-cherished assumptions about practice is difficult and requires great courage, and so it is not surprising that one of the studies in this part (Sarah and Bob's) has been carried out by people who do not fit the definitions of practitioner researchers that we have developed. Perhaps it is sometimes easier to be critical and challenging as an outsider than as an insider.

This is an important point to make, and it is one which is followed up in the final chapter of this book, where we talk about developing criteria for evaluating practitioner research and suggest that one criterion might be the extent to which practitioner research critically examines practice. To do this as an insider, however, requires great clarity and determination as well as a supportive environment in which critical comment is valued rather than feared. For those in the academic world critical comment is a way of life, and for some the fiercer the controversy the better. In the practice world, where the emphasis is perhaps on searching for certainties, controversy can often create anxiety. There is therefore a case for encouraging the critical appraisal of practice, but this must be managed in a way which allows open debate rather than pushes practitioners and researchers into entrenched positions.

CHAPTER 9

Patients' feelings about patients

Debbie Skeil

EDITORS' INTRODUCTION

The following study confounds one of the criticisms or concerns about practitioner research – that it can simply reinforce practitioners' views and assumptions about patient care. The assumption that patients with similar disabilities will derive benefit from contact with each other is one that has long been made in health care, encouraged by movements which seek to value the patients' experience, both within professions and in patient support agencies. This study was initiated by casual observations of events that occurred in practice which seemed to suggest that this was not necessarily the case, and so the researcher decided to investigate these observations in a more systematic way. What she found suggested that, in the case of this patient group at least, contact with others suffering similar health problems could be a frightening and demoralizing experience.

In this way, attentive practice generated a research question and it is important not to underestimate the importance of this contribution. Practice made a contribution to the research in other ways too, namely in the way in which data were collected. As Debbie notes, her skills of taking notes and interviewing patients, which had developed as part of her clinical role, were useful in her conduct and recording of interview data – she had developed the ability to take comprehensive notes in a non-intrusive way, and also the ability to judge the timing and content of her questions. This use of clinical skills in research is an underrated and underacknowledged phenomenon. As practitioners, we spend a great deal of time interacting with patients and clients; some of us develop great interpersonal skills in doing so, whereas others do not. For those who do develop such skills, the conduct of an interview is likely to be easier and more productive than for researchers who have not had such experience and who may not feel comfortable and confident in asking questions. Some practitioner researchers, however, feel anxiety about conducting research interviews, sometimes because they doubt their ability to obtain 'good' data from patients. This fear seems to rest upon the assumption that research interviews are very different to other forms of interview, but it is possible to argue that whereas the type of information asked for may be different, the skills required to obtain it are very similar.

Knowledge and experience of particular patients was also useful in this study, in that it enabled Debbie to adapt her interview style, for example for a lady who had considerable speech problems. This again illustrates the potential value of practitioner experience and knowledge, which is often not explicated in practitioner research. There seems to be an idea that such knowledge is biased or not scientific, in that an outsider researcher would not have these skills and so might obtain different data. This notion seems to originate from notions of science that depersonalize research, in that data can only be regarded as valid if they can be collected by anyone – the person collecting the data should not affect them in any way. As discussed in Chapter 1, this is a very restricting view of the researcher and one which does not allow practitioners to capitalize on and use the skills and knowledge that they have prior to the research, but rather requires them to be denied.

This research also points out one of the potential problems of practitioner research – the possibility that the research might unwittingly exploit the patient–practitioner relationship. As this study was conducted by a doctor, traditionally regarded as a powerful person within any health care setting, there was always the possibility that patients might feel constrained in their responses and fear the possible consequences of giving unwelcome responses. This required the researcher to examine the data carefully to see whether a range of positive and negative comments had been made, a discipline which can be adopted by others who feel that compliance may be a problem. Other strategies could have been used, such as anonymous questionnaires, to reduce the risk of patients feeling constrained by the researcher's practice role, but these may well lead to other problems. There would not only be the practical difficulties of patients with disabilities completing questionnaires without assistance, but also difficulties of interpretation. The interviews were preceded by a general explanation of the purpose of the study and the questions were non-directive, but it is still possible that patients may have mistrusted the explanation, or looked for cues that would tell them what were the right answers. In an interview situation the interviewer can signal verbally and non-verbally that all answers are equally acceptable, and can respond to further questions from the patient. With non-interactive methods of data collection these opportunities do not exist, and there is always the possibility that patients may still try to give the 'right' answers – the difference between a questionnaire and an interview being that in a questionnaire the researcher has no way of judging whether this is the case, or offering further information. Again, this returns us to the interplay between practice and research roles and skills – if practitioners are skilled in developing relationships of trust and acceptance with patients, then their interview data are less likely to reflect patient anxiety about 'acceptable' answers.

Another interesting point about this research is the perception that Debbie has about managerial processes of audit and quality assurance. In contrast to other chapters in this book (for example Chapter 6), where audit processes are seen as inhibitory or conflicting for research, there is a view expressed in this chapter that such processes are healthy stimulants to reflection. Part of the reason for this difference in view may be attributed to the differences in perceived control that practitioners may feel they have over such managerial actions, and it may also be partly due to perceived differences in epistemology. For someone in a position of power, who is a manager, audits may not be viewed as threatening, whereas for those who feel that they have little control over the process they may be seen as potentially damaging exercises. For those whose research methodology contrasts sharply with audit methodology, there may be an additional problem of justifying research approaches. That this does not appear to be the case in this study suggests that conflicts are not always inevitable.

The study in this chapter does have a management orientation in the sense that it is clearly stimulated by the awareness that practice may need to change, and the data are interpreted in this context. The research therefore differs from research done by an outsider with the aims of developing generalized theoretical and academic knowledge, because it is done to develop theoretical understanding, which contributes to practice in a specific context. It would be possible and valuable to develop this study theoretically, for example to say something about concepts of patient self-image and fears of stereotyping, but primarily this research was done to improve and develop practice in a particular setting for a particular client group. This is why the recommendations of this study may seem rather pedestrian – there is no grand theory of patient experience here, but rather a painstaking consideration of changes that might be made in a particular context to improve patient care. This does not necessarily mean that this research does not have relevance to other settings; indeed, it is likely that practitioners working in other settings might find the study generates ideas for improving their care. This is not generalization in the traditional statistical sense, of the type claimed for large studies with random samples and quantitative measures; its usefulness for practitioners rests in the details given about a particular setting which enables readers to identify similarities and differences between the research setting and their own. From this, it then becomes possible for readers to judiciously select those findings that echo their practice and those recommendations which are possible to implement. This seems, in the end, a more meaningful way of using research than the traditional process of generalization.

INTRODUCTION

The main aim of this research project was to ascertain what effect patients who were disabled had on other patients who were disabled. The research setting was a hospital which had quite recently been adapted as a regional neurological rehabilitation centre, but it is housed in the now discontinued Young Disabled Unit (YDU). The YDU was where all the disabled people who could not be found anywhere else to live were put. It became their home and everything was done for them without worrying about trying to help them care for themselves. Many were severely handicapped by physical and cognitive impairments. No further patients will be admitted to the centre to live there.

The rehabilitation inpatients had recently developed a variety of disabilities resulting from neurological insults such as strokes and head injuries. The main process in their rehabilitation is to help them be as independent as can be, minimize their handicap and return them to their previous homes if possible.

There were three wards at the time of the study, one for rehabilitation and respite clients, one for rehabilitation and long-stay clients and one for all long-stay clients. The same dining room was used by everyone, and although there are lots of residents' lounges there is one large sun-lounge that is used by some members of all the wards.

There had been several comments made by patients about their fellow patients. Mainly these had been made by people who were cognitively impaired about others who were also cognitively impaired, e.g. one patient who was slightly verbally aggressive said of another who had a severe memory problem and could also be verbally aggressive: 'When I'm better I'm going to get a shot gun and kill him'.

From my time working on a large spinal injuries unit it seemed that to be surrounded by people with very similar injuries was a great support: the patient in the next bed had just been through the same thing a month ago, and there was always someone worse off than you. So, was it a help or a hindrance having a unit dedicated to serving people with physical and cognitive impairments?

METHODS

There were only 2 months available to collect all the data and write it up, which restricted my choice of research methods. Although I wanted to explore patients' feelings in more depth than a conventional, tightly structured questionnaire would allow, I did not have the time to collect and analyse large amounts of unstructured data. I therefore decided to use semistructured interviews with the patients and to give them only a general description of the study, as I wanted to see whether they would raise the issue of relationships with fellow patients spontaneously. If they did not, I would ask them directly.

The project was agreed to by all heads of departments and the patients' consultants. Each patient was asked if they would be willing to give some of their time for a research project on how people found being at the centre. All the patients had been attending the centre for at least 10 days before I interviewed them, to allow them time to settle in to a very strange environment. All were inpatients, except one who was an inpatient for 36 hours only and was attending the day unit at the time of the interview. The interview was held in a small room away from the ward, where no one could overhear us or was likely to interrupt. I ensured that we both had at least 30 minutes available for the interview.

The first question I asked was: 'How do you find it being at (the centre), not the drugs or the physiotherapy, but being here?' How many more questions were needed varied between patients. I took notes during the interview, having explained that confidentiality would be maintained but that the data would be written up with the names changed. The interview data were supplemented by a book of field notes I recorded of comments made by patients, either to me or passed on by other members of staff while reviewing the patients' progress, and a few pictures illustrating the clustering of patients in rest and recreational areas.

ANALYSIS

I did this by highlighting or underscoring in different colours comments relating to topics that frequently came up in the original notes I made during the interview. The topics I identified were:

- The effect of the patients on the patients – negative and positive;
- The provision of facilities and so-called 'hotel services';
- The effect of mixed-sex wards and bathroom facilities;
- The hospital as a rehabilitation centre; comments that show the difference between an acute hospital and the centre, hence reflecting the philosophy of rehabilitation;
- Compliments;
- Comments relating to the service supplied by therapy/nursing staff;
- Emotions expressed;
- Possible solutions to the problems.

These comments were then put on to the computer under their relevant subject headings, with the patient's identity number and the source of the comment, i.e. interview (i) or field note (f). After printing them out under their relevant headings it was much easier to refer back to them and to analyse them further. The same referencing will be used throughout the report and brief details of the patients can be found in the Appendix to this chapter.

RESULTS

All the patients I asked were quite willing to participate. Some were booked in to see me on their timetable, while others were seen there and then, usually in the late afternoon when most therapy was finished.

The longest interviews were with those who had found the experience most distressing, the average length being 4.75 pages of transcript (about an hour in duration). The three patients who had not found it such a bad experience and had not had previous experience of being with people with physical disability, were all much more difficult to interview, average 2.4 pages and less than half an hour in duration. On reviewing the original transcripts of these patients, 5, 9 and 14, I found that many more questions had to be asked to elicit any response and then the replies were short, despite giving plenty of silence in which any further answers could be given.

The average number of questions for the first page for these three was six, whereas for the distressed patients it was 2.25 for the first page. Patient 4 is the only one to have had previous experience, working for many years with people with physical and cognitive impairments; he talked very freely and was not at all concerned by his fellow patients.

It became very plain to me while doing the interviews that patients find it very traumatic when they first arrive at the centre, and usually take a week or more before getting over the worst of this. The reason for this is the effect of the other patients on them. The greatest distress seemed to be caused by those with not only visible physical disability but also cognitive and/or speech problems. The level of distress caused by this is very significant and led to one lady leaving the hospital within 48 hours of admission. Many of the patients expressed these feelings in their first words in answer to the undirected first question: 'How do you find it being at (the centre)?' Their opening comments include:

13i *Distressing, not prepared for such severely disabled people.*
6i   *When I first arrived I thought it was terrible, I was horrified.*
9i   *Some of the patients, you know, like 2 when he loses his temper, 7 when she screams. I know they are patients but should the mental ones be somewhere else?*

5i   *On the first visit I did not like it much.*
15i   *Hard, I expected folk just like myself, head injury and spinal.*

As I mentioned in the results section, those who found it most distressing talked very freely about it without my even broaching the subject.

None of these people (except 5, who had been an inpatient before) had had any previous experience of people with disabilities. I tried to work out with them just why it was so distressing, and several themes emerged.

A. They did not want to be identified with the disabled patients:
3i   *Just because I have a funny arm (points to shoulder support) and one of them (points to AFO) people must think I am one of them.*

B. They thought they might become like the other disabled patients, or the others might stop them from getting better, or they might never leave the centre:

3i   Q: *Do you think you will become like that?*
      She laughed embarrassingly: *Yes, I worry a lot.*
6i   *I was on the ward with that screaming woman and thought it was an institution . . . I was really horrified, thought I was institutionalized and looked around and thought, "I'm going to be here for the rest of my life" . . . my husband . . . knew it as the institution for incurables.*

C. It was not just sitting in a wheelchair that caused the problem, it was looking abnormal (e.g. drooling, abnormal posture, involuntary movements), speech problems, behavioural problems:

13i   *. . . 17, I didn't think there would be some who could not speak . . . thought people would feed themselves.*

6f   Client 6 was in tears, asking us if she could go home:
      Q: *Can you tell what is upsetting you ?*
6f   *7 was screaming all night, and I didn't get any sleep, my daughter burst into tears yesterday as she was leaving, there is only 8 to talk to, I know she can't help it but with 7 dribbling and screaming I shouldn't be here.*

D. It was distressing seeing such young people disabled, some of whom they identified with their children:

13i   *distressing . . . especially the young people.*

There are too many references to include them all, but in my original report the items relating to the above groups A–D were identified in the margin, and it was clear that the majority of comments were in category C.

Mealtimes came up a few times: no-one spelt out that it was not very easy to watch, but comments included:

13i *When I first came in it was lunch, I was wheeled in and people were being fed . . .*

It was as though it was not socially acceptable to say how horrible it was to watch people make a mess when they eat, or to watch people being fed by others.

Fear was expressed without being broached by the interviewer for several different reasons – some being irrational:

15i *Frightening, know they are harmless, just one of us really . . . some because they could not cope if they were like that themselves:*

15i *Patient 16 can't do anything, that's frightening. If I was like that I could not accept it.*

and some understandably frightened of physical attack :

9i Q: *Why is it frightening?*
He is such a big lad, you don't know what he is about to do next.

So many of these statements relate to the cause of disabled peoples' handicaps, i.e. in the attitude able-bodied persons have towards disabled people, and able-bodied people make up the majority of society. All the interviewees were once able-bodied themselves, and so many of them had those same attitudes.

We hide abnormal people away in special schools, so that few children have ever related to children with any disability. We make it very difficult for people in wheelchairs to get out and about by making our public transport, shops and public buildings inaccessible, and very few people with disabilities can obtain work, even before rising unemployment, so the fear of the unknown is perpetuated into adulthood. None of these people who found the centre distressing had previously had any contact with disabled people. Once they had a chance to see behind the outer shell the fear was removed, as discussed by 13, and they were 'alright'. However, they were able to cope with people with disabilities like their own:

13i *I expected more like myself . . . if someone of the same disability to identify with so would make it easier.*

Presumably the fear has gone if they have the same disability as the other person. They now understand that person's problem, which helps remove the fear, and having experienced the abnormality themselves now realize that it does not affect the person underneath.

It is obviously important to find out why some people can cope and others cannot. The only people who did not find it a bad experience were patients 4, 5 and 14. Patient 4 had worked with similar patients before his current problems; Patient 5 had no noticeable deficit and was admitted for depression, having been an inpatient previously, and

Patient 14 did not find it frightening but instead was encouraged. However, Patient 4 answered to the first question:

I had an idea of what it was like as I go to a centre anyway. To a normal person, well like when I had dinner. . . .

Although he did not spell it out, what he seemed to be saying by his tone of voice and gesturing was that he could cope but many others did not find it so easy.

Patient 9 did not seem to find it quite so distressing as the others, and this was commented on by 6:

6i *others were upset when they first came in, 15 and 9, but it was not so bad as they were put in with us immediately.*

This supports the comments that being surrounded by people with a similar disability is alright, as 9 was admitted into the same bay as 13 and 6. There were other comments that supported this idea, as suggested by 6 above, e.g.:

14i *Now I've seen so many in wheelchairs it makes it easier . . . not the only one . . . feel better . . . some worse than me. . . .*

(he had not had contact with disabled people before).

These comments were reiterated by 9 and 5. The element of support from those with a similar level of disability and the accompanying challenge was raised by 6i:

6i *It is a help if they are similar disabilities. For example, these AFO's we have a good laugh and see who can do it fastest. I can do bras so I'm in demand . . . we laugh about it together. . . .*

This comment was from the same lady who found it *'terrible'* when first admitted, and was made after she was moved into the bay with three other ladies, all with a left-sided weakness (but from different causes).

The patients' own level of disability did not seem to relate to whether they found it distressing or not. Of those who did not find it so distressing, 4 and 5 had been in contact with disabled people before and 5, 9 and 14 are all quieter characters than the others, which is a personal observation from my own and others' contacts with them and is reflected in the length of the interviews.

Patient 5 was very helpful to patients and staff and developed good relationships with people: if anyone needed taking to departments or pushing over to speak to someone he would do that, and many patients and staff commented on how good he was with the patients in doing things for them that they could not do themselves.

14i *5, I know he is a patient but you just have to ask him and he'll do it, we'll miss him when he goes.*

I wanted to find out in the interview why this was. His depression, which had been very severe, lifted amazingly quickly once admitted; was this because he had found a valuable role in life? What made being at the centre such a positive experience? I do not feel that I can confidently extract this from the interview: he gave very brief answers and I had to use very direct questions, but his responses were indicative:

5i   Q: *Why do you push people around in their chairs?*
    no initial answer . . .
    Q: *Do you enjoy it?*
5   *Yes.*
    Q: *Do you do it because you feel you ought to?*
5   *Yes, because I'm walking.*
    Q: *Because you feel you have to or you feel you achieve something doing it?*
5   *Achieve.*

(The above answers are not abbreviated.)

It seems that 5 felt a mixture of obligation and satisfaction in serving his fellow patients. It may be that because of his lack of disability he may not have felt the fear of becoming like them, but rather could appreciate the recovery he had made.

There were several comments that showed the difference between the centre as a rehabilitation centre and an acute hospital. As mentioned previously, one of the main goals is the return to a full role in society, including going home and employment if feasible. This takes some time to achieve, but the process can start in the centre by making it as similar to home as possible, i.e. to dehospitalize things and to make patients as responsible for their actions as is safe. Some of these comments included:

13i   *never came across disabled people before . . . in hospital they are in bed, being nursed.*

These patients had all come from the general hospital, where they were surrounded by disabled people, and yet it only strikes them on coming to the centre that these people are disabled. In the general hospital the patient is encouraged to assume what Schuman (1979) calls the 'dependent patient role'. For example, why is someone who is in hospital expected to wear pyjamas, despite not being in bed? It depersonalizes people, removes their dignity and contributes to the power a doctor has over a patient. At the centre we try to encourage Schuman's rehabilitation stage where 'the patient must learn to live once more in the world of the well'. Everyone is got out of bed in the morning, no matter how disabled they are, sat in a chair (if they need one) in their own clothes and eats in the dining room (if they are able to feed themselves) and the sun-lounge if they cannot. This exposes people's level of disability to everyone: it becomes obvious that someone is being fed because they cannot do it themselves, not because they are too ill to do it. But it is also what a 'normal' person does. The patients are often found in the sun-lounge, which once again exposes their disability to those around.

The area of freedom from rules and freedom to wander, which ties into the philosophy of the unit, was frequently raised e.g.:

4i *Here I can have a meal and a beer, . . . its like a holiday camp . . . at the general it was 2 visitors at a time, here you can have a bus load . . .*

14i *Visitors, there are no restrictions, they can come and go when they like . . .*

6i *There is a lot of leeway in here . . . you can go to the pub and the chip shop . . . when in the general, I thought I would never walk again but now I feel really independent. . . . The attitudes are more positive, it is up to us to do as much as we can. . . .*

DISCUSSION

There have been many examples cited to me in the centre where able-bodied people have found it very upsetting having spent time with disabled people. The effect of disabled people on disabled people can be either positive or negative. Some see others worse than themselves and think how lucky they are; others are terrified of the unknown and worried in case they become like those worse than themselves.

Sadly, our society discriminates against disabled people in many different ways and patients who are newly disabled have grown up in that society with those prejudices, as Carver and Rodda (1978) state about people disabled from birth: 'The impaired person is himself a member of society, learning from childhood the very attitudes that reject him along with his disability'. This makes accepting his disability difficult, and he is challenged further when he cannot accept the disabilities of those who surround him.

There are also very practical issues that will delay the formation of acquaintances that could ease someone settling into the centre. If you are put among a group of strangers in a stressful situation, it is hard enough to strike up conversation. If you cannot move yourself near enough to make conversation easy, and you or your conversant have a speech impediment and all the people are disabled, it is a tall order to expect to settle in easily!

ACTION STEPS

The degree of distress caused to over half the patients interviewed merits a radical review of the current situation. Once it became clear how distressing the centre was to patients, I was able to explore during the interviews how patients thought we might minimize the problem. As a team we have also made plans to implement change to this end. Below are some of the ideas.

We need to think very carefully about the information that is given to patients before they are admitted to the centre, and this was supported by 9i and 15i . Basic information about visiting times and facilities are essential, along with details of what to expect. Already we encourage people and relatives to visit before they are admitted in order to meet staff and reduce the shock on admission, but unfortunately this is not practical for all patients.

The layout of recreational rooms should be reviewed; at present it is a 'them and us' situation, with space available for wheelchairs in the centre and easy chairs in which visitors tend to congregate at the periphery.

The nurses are much busier in the morning and so when someone arrives they may be left a while before being attended to; they suggested that all admissions arrive after 2 p.m., and we did implement this when feasible. As the nurses spend most time with the patients they could introduce a newcomer to other patients, and also broach the subject that many people find it distressing when they first arrive, so giving the patient permission to express his feelings.

The allocation of patients to wards and beds should be carefully reviewed from the social aspect as well as considering therapeutic benefits. As a result of this study we made a major change on the ward that is mixed long-stay and rehabilitation, by moving all the rehabilitation beds together on the ground floor without any long-stay patients being on that floor. This, hopefully, will begin to redress the problem of people thinking they will never leave the centre, as none of the other patients near them have.

All the women should be admitted to a particular bay if possible, to avoid the embarassment suffered by those who find it difficult to live in close proximity to strangers of the opposite sex, and if possible there should always be more than one female inpatient. The mixing of cognitively impaired and intact patients needs to be reviewed and several interviewees thought that they should be separated:

3i   *Those should be away.*
6i   *They should be segregated.*

But it seems that putting those with a similar disability together would be helpful:

6i   Q: *Is it a help or a hindrance being with other people with disabilities?*
      It is a help if they are similar disabilities.

The possibility of an introductory video has been raised – this could perhaps include an overview of the history of the unit, a summary of the people who work there, maybe an introduction to some of the residents and a few words from one of the rehabilitation patients talking about how they found it distressing at first, but how it was eventually a useful stay. This could be shown in the smaller day rooms with a nurse present throughout. This information was requested by 6i and 15i in the Solutions section of the interview.

An informal support group has also been suggested where people could come along for a chat and a cup of coffee, and any problems with settling in can be mulled over and the issue of coping with others' disabilities can be raised. The speech therapists run a communication group to which several people with various communication problems can go. It is a therapeutic group, but they have found that this group (not included in this survey) also find it hard to be with other disabled people. However, once they had been to the group they often enjoyed it. This shows the importance of gentle encouragement to help people overcome their fears, but also the need for enough sensitivity not to subject people to something they cannot cope with and the importance of asking what people want.

When working with people who had had amputations there was a similar response from some of the clients, who did not like seeing others with a higher level of amputation and feared that they too would end up like this. Sometimes there was justification to their fear, but often not. This suggests that if people are placed in this situation, staff need to be sensitive to this area of potential distress, and be prepared to discuss it.

Overall I thought this was a very worthwhile piece of research and its findings were not what I was expecting. I think the use of a semi-structured interview was the most important thing, as it allowed freedom for both the interviewee and the interviewer. I very much hope we will change our policies and then we should repeat the research. However, I do not think we will ever remove all the distress.

PRACTITIONER RESEARCH AS A METHOD

My background is strongly based in the sciences; my introduction to practitioner research and qualitative research came through doing a Master's in Educational Development, which I undertook because of my interest in teaching. I have found many benefits to this form of research that suit my area of work in rehabilitation. This section will be divided into four broad areas: first, a general look at paradigms and research methodologies; secondly, issues related to insider bias; thirdly, some general details important to the method used; and finally, points related to analysis and writing up.

Research paradigms and methodologies

In this section I will try to look at scientific and interpretative paradigms, methodologies used in each and their link with audit and practitioner research. Overall, I found that the difference between the practitioner research that I did and audit and other research I had been involved in, was that practitioner research used an interpretative paradigm and qualitative methods.

The scientific paradigm

Traditional scientific research seeks to establish universal laws that apply to everything. It aims to be objective. A hypothesis is generated to validate a theory and the research aims to test that theory. A typical scientific hypothesis would be: 'This drug controls blood pressure in this patient group with hypertension', and the research would seek to prove this. The method would therefore have to include establishing whether or not the drugs were taken; if they were not, the result would be discarded as not representing the effect of the drug on the blood pressure. The human beings are treated as objects in a controlled setting with regard to their blood pressure. The results are analysed in a quantitative manner using statistics to determine whether or not the results are 'statistically significant'. If they are not, yet more statistical tests are tried and, if they are still not significant, then the theory is disproved.

Clinical audit

Clinical audit was defined by the government as 'the systematic critical analysis of the quality of medical care, including the procedures used for diagnosis and treatment, the use of resources, and the resulting outcome and quality of life for the patient' (Secretary of State, 1989). It was introduced by the government in the late 1980s as a way to monitor the effect of patients' overall clinical management, and is a step away from the controlled environment of the scientific research question. It includes many more aspects of patient management than a pure scientific research question. For example, if the management of blood pressure were audited, questions would include: How is it diagnosed? What investigations then follow? What treatment and follow-up is initiated? Standards are then set and part of the role of audit is asking: How often is this protocol followed (which will include patient compliance)? How successful is the final control of patients' blood pressure? Is the standard reached? The method may measure objective or subjective things, but generally uses statistics and numbers to represent its findings. Scientific research and audit thus concentrate on the management of the *disease* and, as put by Richard Smith (1992): 'Research is concerned with discovering the right thing to do: audit with ensuring that it is done right'.

INTERPRETATIVE PARADIGM

The interpretative paradigm seeks to understand the person and their social situation from the perspective of the respondent. It works on the assumption that human action results from an individual's interpretation of a situation. This involves subjective thoughts and feelings. The researcher has an area of social/psychological dimension he wishes to explore, and from the results a hypothesis is postulated. The researcher is not immune from subjective interpretation of the research project, but this does not mean that the findings are invalid; instead this is described in the method and related to the results. It seeks to illuminate: the results will never be as reproducible as results from a scientific research question; the 'subjects' and 'researchers' have too many subjective variables to be controllable. It may ask questions such as: 'What social factors determine a patient's compliance with the treatment of hypertension?' It may use observation and semistructured interviews to explore the patient's perspective of his management; to find what factors from his background and in his surroundings make him respond in a particular way; to look at his responses to different members of staff. The results will be presented using words and not numbers. They do not have to be statistically significant. An individual's results, even though they may be opposite in nature to all the other results, can still be illuminating with regard to that individual's social and psychological situation.

I would say that practitioner research looks at social, psychological and more subjective aspects of the management of patients who have the diseases that are the concern of scientific research and audit. It uses an interpretative paradigm and a qualitative method to explore and audit the social and psychological aspects of patient care, and the researcher is involved in the patient's care.

AUDIT AND PRACTITIONER RESEARCH

With the advent of audit we have been encouraged to review our working practices to try and improve areas that are found to be deficient and then to repeat the audit of those areas to establish the effect of our improvements. This is very similar to one method used in practitioner research, i.e. the cycle of action research. McNiff (1988) defines this as identifying a problem by reflecting on the situation; imagining a solution; implementing the solution; observing the effects; evaluating the outcomes; modifying actions and ideas from that evaluation; then replanning for the next action step. The one different factor in audit is that the first problem identified is measured and then the solution implemented – it is what you are currently doing, not what you think you are doing. This is why I found the concept of researching one's own work familiar, but the methods used in practitioner research, e.g. semistructured interviews, field notes, are different. By trying to understand how clients perceived the unit, I hoped we could improve the outcome of their treatment. I accepted that social factors within the unit could influence the effect of therapy, and acknowledged that patients' feelings and more subjective factors can be as important as their drug treatments, and can influence their disease management.

QUALITATIVE AND QUANTITATIVE METHODS

A distinctive feature when contrasting quantitative and qualitative methods is that the former respects only numbers, whereas the latter respects words. I find that words have a much greater impact on me than numbers. If you say to me that 60% of clients at the centre ($n = 8$) found parts of their stay very distressing it tells me something, but when words are used it means much more. For example:

13i   *distressing . . . especially the young people.*
3i   *she cried for about an hour on the first night of admission . . . Then her sister arrived and she started crying.*
6i   *When I first arrived here it was terrible, I was horrified. . . .*
15i   *I used to cry in the corner of the sun-lounge.*

Added to this is the impact of facial expressions, intonation and gestures when undertaking the interviews yourself.

Quantitative research accepts only the overall population's results, whereas qualitative research puts equal importance on an individual's results; quantitative researchers are not concerned about answers on the extremes of their range and may discard them as not being representative of the population; qualitative researchers want to know why someone felt this way, because as an individual they do count. It takes some time to realize that both are important. A midwifery tutor summed up people's attitudes to the two approaches when she said that those who use qualitative methods respect both qualitative and quantitative methods, whereas those who use quantitative methods only have little time or respect for qualitative research. When the quantitative approach is 'the baggage you bring with you', it can be hard to accept that maybe qualitative approaches do offer a valid research method. It is even harder to then admit to medical colleagues that you not only believe this but put it into practice! The fear of derision is ever present. Actually writing about it also leaves me feeling vulnerable – scientists do not write about their feelings!

INSIDER BIAS

One argument often raised against practitioner research relates to insider bias. I feel that this bias need not always be a negative one, though. For the negative aspects, I was very aware of the bias that could exist from a doctor interviewing patients which could significantly alter the answers obtained. This comes from two closely linked areas – from the imbalance of power that exists between doctor and patient, and the patient's fear of prejudicing their future treatment by what they say. The traditional 'medical model' places the doctor as controller of the patient's treatment and gives her authority over the patient. Friedson (1970) talks about this power a doctor has as being embodied in the profession of medicine within the order of our society and related to their 'expert' knowledge. Even in a centre that seeks to convert a patient into a client and to give control over their own wellbeing back to the client, the imbalance of power currently remains, largely due to the clients' previous experience of doctor–patient relationships and the present official social order of society.

Secondly, the local provision of NHS services, as it was at the time of the study, meant that clients knew they were unlikely to be able to receive similar treatment outside our unit, and as such would not want to upset the provider (as partly represented by the doctor) of the services they currently needed. For both reasons it may therefore be difficult for a client to comment to a doctor negatively on a situation they feel the doctor to be a part of. It may be easier to comment on the food than on nursing or medical care. As a matter of interest, one client did talk of her negative experiences with a doctor when I asked her directly why she had been upset.

However, the effect of this negative bias can also exist in quantitative methods, particularly where they seek to measure subjective issues, as in a survey of outpatients and their views on the service they receive. Awareness of this highlights the care that is needed in testing the validity of any method that measures, either quantitatively or qualitatively, something subjective. Does the patient answer the question by saying how he really feels, or how he thinks it prudent or socially acceptable to answer? Whether people feel able to talk about issues related to their treatment will depend on what is socially acceptable, which in turn relates partly to the individual's social background. For example, some people from northern England are blunter in what they say than southerners (personal observation of a southerner who now lives up north!). Some individuals feel able to tell you exactly what they think about everything, good and bad, while others would not complain about anything; some underplay their problems, others overplay them.

When testing reliability similar care is needed – if testing interobserver reliability the use of two doctors using an interview technique may give similar results. However, if a doctor and an outsider, both suitably experienced in the technique, administer the same method you may get very different results but biases still remain – the outsider researcher may still be perceived as having authority over the subject and social restraints which relate to this will remain. Conversely, the doctor may gain more information because of that insider bias; this will be discussed later.

If none of the patients had said anything bad about the unit I would have had to conclude either that we ran a perfect unit or, more likely, that I should not trust the findings of my research: that the insider bias meant that clients did not feel able to talk to me about these things. The fact that patients did talk about good and bad aspects of their stay suggests that this was not the major problem I thought it would be. The negative responses indicated that some of the patients were answering honestly. It may be that they would have said more to an outsider, but they might not have done.

On the positive side, insider bias might have contributed to some of the answers I received, for at least four reasons. First, it is often easier to talk to someone you know than to a stranger, and all these patients knew me already. They had already been able to judge how much they could trust me. Secondly, I also knew them; I knew their characters a little, and their social background. I knew the way they behaved and related to others outside the interview situation. I had been able to judge the best way to communicate with each individual, and hopefully to get the most out of the interview because of this. I knew that the three who were very quiet when I interviewed them were also very quiet the rest of the time, and not just with the doctors. This advantage of insider research also means that if an individual tells you one thing, but everything you see of them at times outside the interview indicates something contrary, you should doubt the reliability of that individual's interview. Thus insider knowledge helped me judge whether or not my interview was valid, but in a way that cannot be quantified. An outsider will not have that knowledge available to them.

Thirdly, we shared a common knowledge of the unit, the other patients and how they behaved and a basic understanding of how the unit ran. This knowledge could thus be taken for granted during the interview. The patients did not have to spell out some of the things or people that were troubling them, they could mention a name and know that I would know them also. For example:

13i   . . . I was wheeled in at lunchtime.

Although the tone of voice displayed her dismay, she said no more and did not need to, as she knew I knew what lunchtime was like – lots of people being fed, dribbling and messy. It is socially much easier to imply 'unspeakable' things than to have to describe in full what upset you, and hence I feel that the shared knowledge facilitated the interviews. Obviously a researcher using an interpretative method who decided to work within the unit to overcome these problems (Webb, 1992), and especially someone with a paramedical background, would also understand some of these things, but the more inside a system you become the more like insider research it becomes.

Fourthly, by being an insider I knew the impairments each of these patients had, and my medical background meant that I appreciated how this affected their life and especially their ability to communicate. Although an outsider would have to ask permission and could begin to understand the problems by talking to a member of staff, it would not be first-hand knowledge. A sociologist undertaking such research would not have understood the effect of the impairment on the individuals. The more reading and enquiring a sociologist did to understand these problems, again the more like a practitioner researcher he would become.

My insider knowledge thus affected how I interviewed patients because of my knowledge of their impairments. The interview style was altered for client 3 and almost certainly contributed positively to the value of the interview. Client 3 had an expressive dysphasia and had problems finding her words. I knew that I needed to give her plenty of time to answer and that she might need words or letters suggested to her to help her finish a sentence. I did do this during the interview and she would keep rejecting ideas until I suggested the one she wanted. A non-practitioner might not realize that such tactics were necessary, and could feel it was answering for the client. However, the continued rejection of inappropriate answers, frustration shown until the right answer was found and knowledge that without such an approach no answer (and much agony for the client) would have resulted show how the insider knowledge of the treatment approaches used with that client facilitated the interview. I also knew that slow, short sentences were a result of her aphasia and not due to a low IQ, shyness or fear.

INSIDER RESEARCH – EFFECTS ON METHODS

Being a doctor interviewing patients my choice of method was biased. We are constantly interviewing people to elicit their problems and then recording the data in written format for us and others to review later. As such, I will probably be more accurate using an interview technique and notes than someone who does not do this daily. Many would say that ideally a tape-recording should be used, or video. I was not keen for several reasons: first, it might have inhibited both the clients and me; secondly, the practical difficulties of transcribing the recording; and thirdly I was concerned about possible medicolegal implications.

My medical knowledge also affected my choice of interviewees, but for humane reasons. I excluded two patients who were severely depressed. Although I acknowledged that being at the centre might have contributed to their depression, I was concerned that the interview could have been further detrimental to their mental state.

One final area that I noticed as being fundamentally different between an external researcher and a practitioner researcher is the breadth of interest the researcher has in the unit, and the impact this has on the method used and the data collected. An external researcher will have a clearly defined question to answer and will probably be interested in little else. However, if you work in the place and are committed to striving towards better care for your patients, your interest embraces anything that will do that. If a very structured interview is used you will probably only receive the answers to the questions you ask, which might not be the questions the client would like you to ask. If your concern is to improve the unit, rather than to produce a report on a research project, you will design the method accordingly. This is the advantage I found of the semistructured interview: it allowed the client freedom to talk about what was important to them, rather than what I thought was important when I designed my questions. It also allowed me to pick up on the way things were said, together with non-verbal cues, and gave me freedom to pursue them (Wragg, 1982). For example, if during an interview the patient told me the food was awful, I did not dismiss it as irrelevant to my research questions: 'How do disabled people affect disabled people?' I was interested in it because it was relevant to my clients' overall wellbeing. This influences the breadth of the research question I asked and of the data I recorded. Everything depends on the aim of your research, and so it is important to be clear about this at the beginning. You need not use all your data when writing up your research, but it may be important to your everyday practice. It is better to record too much and not to use all of it, and it is essential to record enough to answer your research question!

INSIDER RESEARCH – IMPACT OF THE STUDY

I feel that practitioner research for research's sake is futile. Practitioner research, like audit, should improve our clients' management. However, there is another benefit to be gained from insider research in the effect it may have on the researcher. Doing research on your work is a time-consuming occupation, but because you have heard it 'from the horse's mouth', and handle the data so much, the exercise has a much greater impact on you than just reading the report in a journal. You take the results more seriously because it is not so easy to brush aside or forget the faces, voices and words you have seen and heard, and actions to correct the problems are more likely to follow. I would also hope that the research might have a similar impact on others, both within and outside the unit. Although it will not be as profound as the first-hand experience, it may still be more effective because it is a professional colleague who understands their work situation (rather than if it was an outsider doing the study).

WRITING UP

One interesting thing I and others have noticed is that memory is an important adjunct to recording data. When I wrote up the report I only looked at the scripts to quote what someone said: I knew roughly everything that had been said, and by taking notes it had been ingrained in my memory. When writing any findings, to be rigorous in what you do it is important not to record anything purely from memory without indicating this in the report. This allows those reading it to weight its relevance accordingly. With any research the findings are only as reliable as the method used, and a detailed account of the method is essential if people are to be able to judge it.

At the end of the day, if you write up your study adequately other health care professionals should be able to judge for themselves whether or not a piece of practitioner research is useful by studying the details of the method used. If the method is flawed, the results will be flawed. It is vital that the explanation of method, subjects, researchers and their background, how the interviews were done etc. is not neglected when writing up. People can then judge the results for themselves. For those interested in further analysing different aspects of the data or undertaking an analytical survey, the case data, as described by Stenhouse (1978), although bulky, are still available for people to see.

CONCLUSION

The practitioner research I undertook revealed areas of stress that some of the clients at the centre were exposed to that I had not been aware of prior to the research, and which the clients had not talked about. We are now very aware that some of our disabled patients find other disabled patients very distressing; it is freely talked about with clients; it is frequently recognized as a major problem for large numbers of our clients and their families; and, within the unit, we are trying to reduce the level of distress it does cause. Although there were concerns about the method used and the bias introduced by a doctor interviewing her clients, I feel that the insider bias benefited the research considerably. I am convinced that the results have credibility and auditability (Guba and Lincoln, 1981): they have certainly been found to be reliable as far as my encounters with clients since then have been concerned.

APPENDIX

Brief description of patients referred to in the text and their disabilities.

1. Rehabilitation client. Female, 50s. Severe problems understanding language and cannot consistently say yes or no. Also right-sided weakness. Can walk.
2. Rehabilitation client. Male, 20s. Head injury. Aggressive verbal outbursts. Full-time wheelchair user at present, coordination problems in arms and legs. Slurred speech. Cognitively reasonable.
3. Rehabilitation client. Female, 50s. Right-sided weakness. Moderate problems in word finding and tends to use very short, not fully structured sentences. No cause found for stroke. Can walk.
4. Rehabilitation client. Male, 30s. Non-traumatic spinal cord damage. Lifelong physical disability. In wheelchair.
5. Rehabilitation client. Male, 20s. Head injury. Minimal deficit. Hearing loss since childhood. Walks easily.
6. Rehabilitation client. Female, 40s. Left-sided weakness. No speech problems. Initially in wheelchair.
7. Long-term resident. Female, 50s. Cerebral palsy. No speech. No ability to care for herself. In wheelchair. Screams a lot.
8. Long-term resident. Female, 60s. Minimal one-sided weakness, mostly now better. Able to look after herself. Can walk. Often uses wheelchair.
9. Rehabilitation client. Female, 50s. Left-sided weakness. No speech problems. Was in wheelchair at time of interview.
10. Rehabilitation client. Male, 50s. All four limbs weak. Wheelchair. Speech not bad.
11. Long-term resident. Male, 60s. Had a stroke, now recovered. Mild lifelong learning difficulties.
12. Rehabilitation client. Male, 30s. Head injury. Slurred speech. Right-sided weakness, wheelchair, disinhibited. Abnormal posture right arm.
13. Rehabilitation client. Female, 50s. Left-sided weakness, no speech problems. Was in wheelchair at time of interview.
14. Rehabilitation client. Male, 60s. Unable to use arms or legs normally. Spinal cord injury. In wheelchair.

15. Rehabilitation client. Male, 30s. Spinal cord injury. Almost walking.
16. Long-term resident. Male, 50s. No movement of any limbs. No speech. Lacks facial expression. Electric chair with chin-controlled scanning device.
17. Rehabilitation client. Male, 20s. Head injury. Severe speech problems, few words. Left-sided weakness. Wheelchair. Drools. Abnormal posture left arm.
18. Respite. Male, 50s. Rare muscle disease. Weakness of all four limbs. Overnight ventilator (needs tube going into windpipe for this which is there permanently).
19. Rehabilitation client. Male, 40s. Head injury. No speech. Limited use of limbs. Wheelchair. Not aware of what is going on. Large scar on head.
20. Rehabilitation client. Male, 50s. Left-sided weakness. Severe perceptual problems. Some speech problems.
21. Long-term resident. Male, 60s. Wheelchair. Behavioural problems. Limited range of words. Abnormal-looking left arm.
22. Rehabilitation client. Female, 20s. Poor coordination of all limbs, rapidly improving. Slight speech problems.

REFERENCES

Carver, V. and Rodda, M. (1978) *Disability and the Environment*, Elek, London.
Friedson, E. (1970) *Profession of Medicine: a Study of the Sociology of Applied Knowledge*, Dodd, Mead and Co., New York.
Guba, E.G. and Lincoln J.S. (1981) *Effective Evaluation*, Jossey-Bass, San Francisco.
McNiff, J. (1988) Making sense of the data, in *Action Research: Principles and Practice*, (ed J. McNiff), Macmillan, London, pp. 73–87.
Schuman, E. A. (1979) Stages of illness and medical care, in *Patients, Physicians and Illness*, (ed E. G. Jaco), Free Press, New York, pp. 145–61.
Secretary of State for Health, Wales, Northern Ireland and Scotland (1989) *Medical Audit. Working Paper 6*, HMSO, London.
Smith, R. (1992) Audit and research. *British Medical Journal*, **305**, 905–6.
Stenhouse, L. (1978) Case study and case records: towards a contemporary history of education. *British Educational Research Journal*, **4**(2), 21–39.
Webb, C. (1992) The use of first person in academic writing: objectivity, language and gatekeeping. *Journal of Advanced Nursing*, **17**, 747–52.
Wragg, E.C. (1982) Conducting and analysing interviews, in *Guides in Educational Research*, (ed M.B Youngman), Nottingham University, TRC, England pp.177–97.

CHAPTER 10

How adults with learning difficulties and their informal carers perceive professional practice

Bob Heyman and Sarah Huckle

EDITORS' INTRODUCTION

The following chapter provides a useful contrast to the previous chapters as it focuses on the client's rather than the practitioner's perspective. This book has argued the case for developing practitioner research. In the first section it was noted that practitioner research appears to be about *improvement*. This raises the question of improvement for whom and under what circumstances. Clearly, pursuing practitioner research for its own sake may well become a forum for validating professional rhetoric. Indeed, avoiding this is one of the biggest issues confronting many practitioners when they embark on a research project.

This chapter indicates how clients' views can provide a useful counterbalance to professional rhetoric by providing data which challenges some of the cherished ideals held by the professionals. Moving outside the professional arena and eliciting the views of clients can provide the opportunity to introduce a critical discourse to a research project where the researcher is experiencing difficulties in going beyond the taken-for-granted assumptions of the professionals. For instance, Bob Heyman and Sarah Huckle's data highlight the tensions that exist between the formal carers' perceptions of the role of the adult training centre, which was to promote independence, and the perceptions of the clients' informal carers or parents, who viewed the centre as a 'safe haven' for their offspring. More importantly the data graphically illustrate the rigidity in the current provision of care which prevents clients and their parents taking risks and moving out of the centre, as it may be very difficult for them to regain a place should they wish to return in the future.

This illustrates how, without discussions with informal carers, the formal practitioners can make assumptions about the attitudes of the informal carers which may be mistaken. In reality the informal carer's views are derived in part from the rigidity of the service offered. This highlights an incongruity between the stated goals of the formal carers or practitioners, which was the promotion of independence for the client, and the structure of the service offered which militated against the fulfilment of this goal. The chapter indicates the need for practitioners to reconsider the structure of the service offered to clients if congruence is to be achieved between their espoused goals and the service they offer. It is unlikely that incongruity would become apparent without taking into account the views of clients and their informal carers.

At another level the chapter raises the issue of whether practitioner research can ever really reflect the client's perspective. There is an inherent tension between the expertise of professionals, which has been selectively developed to meet needs defined as legitimate by service providers, and the clients' own definition of their needs. It is clear from this chapter that the practitioners interpreted service provision in terms of therapeutic objectives. This serves two purposes: first, it provides a basis for developing skills and expertise within the labour market of health care; secondly, it provides a rationale for demanding the continued funding of the service.

However, it was apparent that many of the informal carers or parents viewed the centre as a 'safe haven' in a potentially hostile world. The centre was valued because it allowed the client to assume the pattern of a normal adult life without its attendant risks and responsibilities. Although it may be possible to make a strong case for providing this type of service from a social or ethical perspective, it falls outside the current rhetoric of provision and therefore is unlikely to be provided on these grounds alone. This raises the issue of power and control in the provision of services and highlights how pursuing research from the client's perspective may identify needs which are not considered to be the legitimate concern of service providers.

INTRODUCTION

This chapter discusses some of the data from a qualitative study of the views of adults with relatively mild learning difficulties living with relatives and attending adult training centres (ATCs). The methodology is summarized briefly in the next section. Adults' views are compared with those of their informal and formal carers. The core category

(Strauss and Corbin, 1990, pp. 123–4) which emerged from the data, around which analysis was organized was the management of perceived hazards by adults, informal and formal carers (Heyman and Huckle, 1993a,b).

There was evidence throughout our research data of a tension between, on the one hand, the desire of adults, informal and formal carers for the adults to develop lifestyles which were as 'normal' as possible (Wolfensberger, 1983) and, on the other hand, the need to protect them from perceived dangers. This tension was found across the whole range of activities that adults might undertake independently of carers, including everyday living skills such as cooking or using sharp knives, going out alone in the local community, getting a job, living independently, extending friendships outside the ATC and developing sexual relationships.

The ways in which adults coped with the dilemma of hazards could be understood as part of a family dynamic which, in most cases, could be placed into one of three categories. The most common, 'shared danger avoidance', characterized the approach to hazards of 11 of the 20 families included in our sample. In these families, adults and informal carers adopted a safety-first policy and developed a lifestyle for the adult which was family- centred, apart from daily 'work' at the ATC. For example, adults and informal carers agreed that it was too dangerous for the adult to go out alone in the local community.

A second group of seven families seemed to take a 'limited risk' approach to coping with hazards. The adults were able to go out alone, meet friends outside the ATC and meet their boy or girlfriend without a chaperon. Informal carers expressed some anxiety about these activities but calculated that the benefits to the adult outweighed the risks. The activities were often hedged with restrictions designed to reduce risk, for example requiring the adult to be home fairly early in the evening, or to be accompanied back home, and the area in which risk-taking was permitted was mostly limited to activities normal for a child living in the parental home. Adults and informal carers in this group largely ruled out the possibility of the adult living independently, getting a job, leaving the ATC, developing a sexual relationship or getting married.

In two families there was overt conflict between an adult man and his family, with the adult wanting to live independently, get a job and get married, whereas the parents ruled out these activities. In these families, in contrast to those in which limited risk-taking was accepted, the adults wanted to exit from the boundaries of the family and to develop away from a childlike role.

A similar threefold classification was developed by Winik, Zetlin and Kaufman (1985) on the basis of qualitative research in the USA. Our classification proved to have good interrater reliability and was closely associated with the social characteristics of the families. Families in the 'limited risk-taking' group were likely to have low socioeconomic status and to have a single main informal carer (for example because the parents had been divorced).

Two explanations for this relationship can be suggested. First, poorer families and those with a single informal carer may have had to become more risk-tolerant because they did not have the human or material resources to be more protective. Secondly, there may be cultural differences associated with social class affecting attitudes to the adults taking risks. Middle-class parents, as a group, appear to evaluate the abilities of their own children with learning difficulties more negatively (Iano, 1970). More speculatively, middle-class culture may be generally less risk-tolerant. The result, perhaps ironically, was that the poorer families had attitudes towards risk-taking and normalisation which were closer than those of middle-class families to the attitudes of formal carers at the ATC, since the latter favoured risk-taking and normalization.

Any scheme classifying complex processes of social adaptation into a small number of ideal types has to be treated with caution. Several limitations of our scheme must be pointed out. First, one or two families were near the borderline between 'danger avoidance' and 'risk-taking', and so hard to classify. The researchers decided, somewhat arbitrarily, that families would be categorized as risk-taking if the adult could move around the local community to a variety of destinations without being accompanied by a carer. Secondly, family dynamics were not static. One middle-class family did a marked 'flip' from danger avoidance to limited risk-taking about a year after being interviewed. This suggests that the relationship between socioeconomic status and approaches to risk-taking which we identified may itself be a temporary product of particular historical circumstances.

Thirdly, the finding that risk-taking was, at most, limited probably reflects sampling limitations rather than inherent parental or adult conservatism. Our sample was confined to more able adults attending ATCs, a marginal group with respect to their ability to lead a normal life. Families with more risk-tolerant attitudes may act in ways that prevent adults from being segregated in the first place, although little is known about the processes that lead to a person being labelled as having a learning difficulty.

Fourthly, although adults in the 'shared danger avoidance' group agreed that the community was a dangerous place, it was not the case that they were content with a life which revolved round the parental family and ATC. As the interviewer got to know them through repeated encounters, all the adults in this group revealed frustration, the most common source being inability to meet friends from the ATC outside this setting. A number of studies of the views of adults with learning difficulties living at home have documented the constraints that adults feel (e.g. Flynn and Saleem, 1986; Richardson and Richie, 1989).

However, in our research adults in the 'limited risk-taking' group did not experience the same level of frustration because they were able to move relatively freely around the local community. This suggests that it is necessary to differentiate the experience of adults with learning difficulties living at home.

This chapter discusses one part of our data which has some relevance to practice development, and focuses on the following questions: How did adults, informal carers and formal carers view the ATC? and How far can the views of these 'stakeholders' be understood in terms of their ways of coping with hazards?

Implicit in our selection of these questions is the view that user perspectives provide an important source of information for practice development (Heyman and Huckle, 1994). Two related reasons why user perspectives are particularly important in the present context can be given. First, there appears to be a considerable gap between formal carers' views of the ATC as a normalizing agency and adult perceptions of it as constraining. The gap is, perhaps, sharpest in relation to attitudes towards sexual relationships (Johnson and Davies, 1989). Secondly, skills learnt at the ATC (e.g. cooking) are often not applied at home because of a lack of coordination between the ATC and informal carers (Cathermole, Jahoda and Markova, 1987). Formal carers tend not to see the whole picture, whereas adults naturally take a holistic view because they are the only people fully exposed to their own lives.

METHODS

Analysis, primarily qualitative, was carried out of interviews with 20 adults, 10 male and 10 female, aged 19–35, who attended two ATCs in an urban area of northeast England and so were socially labelled as having learning difficulties. The area in which they lived is characterized by high levels of unemployment and social deprivation, but has pockets of middle-class affluence. Nineteen adults lived with one or both parents and one lived with a sibling. The criteria for inclusion in the sample were that the adult should attend one of the two ATCs and be able to communicate well enough to be interviewed. The sample represented the upper ability range of those attending the ATCs and included all but four or five eligible adults who were excluded for reasons of availability and convenience. For each adult, at least one informal carer was interviewed. The interviewer (SH) kept a diary and noted the views of formal carers at the ATC. Eight interviews were conducted with formal carers at the ATCs after the data on 'user' views had been collected and analysed. All persons who were approached agreed to participate.

Adults were interviewed over several sessions at the ATC, informal carers over one session in their homes and formal carers over one session at the ATC. All interviews were carried out in a setting where they could not be overheard and confidentiality was guaranteed. Total interview times ranged between 6 and 9 hours for adults, 3–6 hours for informal carers and 1–2 hours for formal carers. The interviewer visited the ATC on four occasions before interviewing commenced in order to establish rapport. Interview questions were open-ended in order to minimize acquiescence (Sigelman *et al.*, 1986) with funnelling techniques used to cover any areas which had been omitted. Adults were encouraged to express their own opinions about sensitive topics, e.g. sexual relationships. More personal areas were only raised after trust had been established. Care was taken to ensure that adults fully understood the purpose of the interview.

Interviews with adults and informal carers were semistructured around standard questions in the following areas: leisure, employment, education, friendship, relationships with the opposite sex, relationships at home and prospects for the future. The main focus in the adult interviews was on their own views, but they were also asked about the views of informal carers. Interviews with informal carers focused mainly on how they saw the adult's views, needs and capabilities. There were some additional questions concerning their own needs and feelings, e.g. how they would feel if the adult left home.

Information about the views of formal carers at the two ATCs was obtained from a convenience sample of eight formal carers, including the managers of the ATCs, four senior care officers and two care assistants. The interviews covered adult capability and need for independence, hazards, attitudes of informal carers and relationships between formal and informal carers.

ADULTS' EXPLANATIONS FOR BEING AT THE ATC

Formal carers at the ATC saw their role in terms of normalization, encouraging adults to develop everyday living skills which would enable them to live more independent lives. But the adults did not, on the whole, see things this way. Underlying their own explanations of why they were at the ATC was a view of themselves as 'not handicapped'. There was a hermeneutic problem in that we were unable to use the politically correct term 'learning difficulties' with adults, as they were completely unfamiliar with it.

INTERVIEWER *Do you think you are mentally handicapped?*
ADULT *Not really.*
INTERVIEWER *Why?*
ADULT *I can walk and they can't.*
INTERVIEWER *Why do you think you come to the centre?*
ADULT *To work.*

This kind of response was the most common. One explanation is that adults maintained their self-esteem by rejecting the stigmatizing label of mental handicap. They also maintained self-esteem by applying this label to other adults at the ATC who had a greater degree of disability than themselves. As a result, they were reluctant to see themselves as coming to the ATC to learn, since to them this would have meant that they were indeed handicapped. The difficulty adults had with the stigmatizing label 'handicapped' and the resulting problems in explaining why they were at the centre are illustrated by the following:

INTERVIEWER *Why do you think you go to the centre?*
ADULT *(Pause) I went to —— special school before I came here.*
INTERVIEWER *Why do you think you went to a special school and why do you think you came here?*
ADULT *I don't know . . .*
INTERVIEWER *Do you think you are handicapped?*
ADULT *A bit handicapped.*

One adult defined herself as 'mentally handicapped' and also, exceptionally, viewed the functions of the ATC in terms consistent with normalization. Her definition of 'mental handicap' was consistent with the explanation given by her parents as to why she was at the ATC. It illustrates the difficulty of mapping the *social category* of attending an ATC on to *properties of the individual* such as 'mental handicap'.

INTERVIEWER *Do you think you are mentally handicapped?*
ADULT *Yes.*
INTERVIEWER *Why?*
ADULT *Brain damage. I take fits . . .*
INTERVIEWER *Why do you think you come to the centre?*
ADULT *To learn things.*

One adult had a financial explanation of why she was at the ATC:

INTERVIEWER *Why do you think that you are in the centre?*
ADULT *I don't know. Since I was 16 I have been coming here . . . I said to my mum shall I get a job? and she said no. If I got a job and I didn't like it I couldn't come back here and my money would stop. My mum needs the money because she is under the doctor like.*

This explanation was one advanced by formal carers at the ATC, who believed that some informal carers were financially motivated to prevent their children becoming more independent and leaving the ATC. Most informal carers denied that they were financially motivated, but some expressed a fear that if their child left the ATC, e.g. for a sheltered workshop, and things did not work out, the child would not be able to return to the ATC.

ADULT ATTITUDES TO FORMAL CARERS

We identified three important themes in adults' views of formal carers: first, a view of formal carers as friends; secondly, expressions of dependency on formal carers; and thirdly, a variety of more or less rebellious attitudes to formal carers as authority figures.

Formal carers as friends

About two-thirds of the informal carers believed that the adults were indiscriminately friendly and not capable of developing special attachments. The tendency of adults to describe trainers as friends was perhaps associated with this belief. However, our interview material shows that nearly all of the adults did have special friendships and could clearly distinguish between close and ordinary friends.

The adults' tendency to describe formal carers as friends arose more from unfilled need and lack of opportunities to develop new relationships than from 'mental handicap', as illustrated below.

INTERVIEWER *How do you get on with the people at college?*
ADULT *Some of them nice, some cruel.*
INTERVIEWER *How are they cruel?*
ADULT *They tell you off and I don't like it.*
INTERVIEWER *Have you made any new friends at college?*
ADULT *Yes.*
INTERVIEWER *Who?*
ADULT *One of the teachers.*

Dependency on formal carers

More than half the adults felt that they could not venture out into the local community on their own and therefore saw staff as a necessary protection. The quote below illustrates the pressures adults are put under, e.g. by informal carers, in order to protect them from danger.

INTERVIEWER *Would you like to be able to go out on your own?*
ADULT *I don't like going out on my own. I like someone there with me.*
INTERVIEWER *You do?*
ADULT *So there is someone there to keep an eye on you so that you keep out of mischief . . . I like going out in groups with a member of staff. I like doing that because I can talk to people.*

Rebellion

On the other hand, the staff were often seen as 'big brother', depriving adults of their autonomy:

> INTERVIEWER *Are there any other things you like to do (at the ATC)?*
> ADULT *I want to be my own boss. When I am in here I want to be my own boss, but the staff always tell me what to do.*

Problems of autonomy versus control occurred most frequently in connection with sexual relationships. Most of the adults had a boy or girlfriend at the ATC but only a small number were able to see this person outside the ATC. The adults had had it drummed into them that anything other than mild kissing and cuddling was 'rude', and were clearly torn between their own needs and the messages they had received that sexual relationships were wrong. The quotation below illustrates the difficulty of distinguishing between the 'voice' of the adults and the 'voices' of those who have told them what to think.

> INTERVIEWER *Would you ever like to go on a trip with —— (girlfriend) with no staff with you?*
> ADULT *think I would sometimes, but I think it is better to have staff with us, to be honest.*
> INTERVIEWER *Why do you think that?*
> ADULT *With staff you know you are doing the right thing.*
> INTERVIEWER *Why do the staff make you do the right thing?*
> ADULT *. . . If you are courting somebody there has to be a chaperone there.*
> INTERVIEWER *Why?*
> ADULT *Because I am always putting my arm around her a lot . . .*
> INTERVIEWER *Are there any things that you would like to do with —— that you can't do?*
> ADULT *I am alright with ——. But on the other hand I would say different. I would like to cuddle her more. I would like to be closer to her.*

Two of the adult men rejected the ATC entirely and expressed a strong wish to leave, to obtain employment and to live independently of their parents. However, their parents would not 'allow' them to do this. One of these adults described an 'escape from Colditz' experience while on a group holiday with other adults:

> ADULT *You're supposed to not go out of the gates, and I did the funniest thing in my life. We went to —— one year and we had to wear this badge, a green badge that shows you are a trainee. So the first thing that I did was to take it off. I went up the gardens, behind the gates. This man turned round and said, "Can I help you sir?". I said, "Yes you can". He says, "Are you a trainee or are you staff?". I said, a bit cool, "I'm staff. I've come on holiday with my centre taking some of the trainees on*

holiday". I said, "I'm going out to get some stuff". He was trying to find out if I was handicapped or not. He let me out.

ADULT UNDERSTANDING OF 'TRAINING'

Adults received a variety of training programmes, both in the ATC and at further education colleges in areas such as activities of daily living, road safety and literacy. The colleges were almost universally popular, partly because they were 'normal' institutions, although social mixing with people from outside the ATC was minimal.

> INTERVIEWER *Are you at college or involved in education?*
> ADULT *I'm in a self help group . . .*
> INTERVIEWER *Are the people at college mentally handicapped?*
> ADULT *I go with the mentally handicapped.*
> INTERVIEWER *Do you like going to college?*
> ADULT *I feel like normal.*

For training to effectively increase autonomy it needs to be sustained, applied in the world outside training and supported by the community, particularly informal carers. Adults reported occasional successes, e.g. learning to use public transport and being able to use it regularly, but in most cases training had little impact on everyday life. One problem was adults' fear that an activity such as going out alone was too dangerous or beyond their capabilities. Other problems were lack of continuity in training and failure to obtain the support of informal carers.

Lack of continuity in training had a devastating impact on both adults and informal carers. For example, one adult had worked on a special work scheme operated by the local council. His parents, who were clearly 'minimal risk takers' had, with some anxiety, allowed him to participate and even to get a bus to work on his own.

> INTERVIEWER *Did he enjoy working on the [work] scheme?*
> INFORMAL CARER *He liked it. We were very dubious. It was about 11 years ago . . . It is the parents who think they can't do it – they hold them back. We are aware that they are very vulnerable. We protect them and tend to be over the top . . . He had to learn to travel on his own which was a worry.*

The learning experience was as much for the informal carers as for the adult, and this example illustrates clearly the need to avoid locating 'learning difficulty' solely in the disability of the adult. The scheme folded after 2 months and the adult was currently 'unable' to use public transport. He remembered having had a job, 11 years ago, and indicated that he preferred it to being in the centre.

The next quotation illustrates how adults could be seriously hurt through lack of continuity in care.

INTERVIEWER *Has she ever been out with a volunteer?*

INFORMAL CARER *A long time ago a girl from an organization used to come round one night a week and take her to Hebburn community centre and talk to her. It lasted for three or four months and —— really enjoyed it then the girl left the service.*

—— was very upset when she stopped coming, and she would talk about her for a long time afterwards, and if they were going to find someone else. Even now she will talk about it now. You see —— got used to the routine of someone coming, and it breaks their faith when it stops.

Sex education was a particular minefield. Adults' knowledge about sexual intercourse, pregnancy, abortion, AIDS etc. was quite high, but the adults said that they had acquired little of this information from formal sex education. The main sources they reported were television, other adults and pornographic material (e.g. films discovered in their parents' wardrobes and watched in secret). Informal carers were ambivalent about or opposed to adults receiving sex education. Some felt that it was needed but most felt either that the adult they were caring for was not interested in sexual matters or that sex education would encourage the adult and lead to irresponsible behaviour. Formal carers, in contrast, felt that adults were capable of responsible sexual behaviour if they were given appropriate information and guidance.

INFORMAL CARER PERSPECTIVES

Attending the ATC was a mainly enjoyable activity for adults, providing their main outlet outside the family for social contacts, recreational and work activities. However, their experiences, when viewed from their perspective, appeared to be doing little to promote normalization, independence or autonomy. One reason commonly put forward for adult dependency is that parents and other informal carers are overprotective and hold their offspring back from achieving their full potential. The formal carers in the ATCs certainly expressed this view.

Labelling informal carers as overprotective does not help us to understand how they viewed the ATC. As with the adults, we need to make sense of a diversity of points of view. However, there were some important similarities in the ways in which informal carers saw the future trajectory of the adults, and therefore the role of the ATC. First, they believed that the adult would and should live with the informal carer as long as possible, eventually being passed to other relatives or into residential care. Secondly, they saw the ATC as a permanent safe refuge and outlet for the adult. Thirdly, they expressed doubts about the quality of life for the adult which would result from alternatives to living with informal carers and attending the ATC. Fourthly, they believed that the adult had, on the whole, achieved his or her potential and were not particularly concerned about the acquisition of new skills. There was evidence of a cultural divide, with some informal carers seeing formal carers as pushing the adults beyond the level of which they were capable, sometimes for reasons of administrative convenience. The two quotations below illustrate some of these themes.

> INFORMAL CARER *I don't know why but they had ——'s name down to go into residential care. They said they would love to have ——. But they didn't have television, the things that —— needs, and were very strong on religion. What was the point of putting —— in there when she doesn't understand religion, and it would be unfair to be put in a place where she might see herself as handicapped.*
>
> INFORMAL CARER *We got a letter asking if —— would like to go in the laundry and I said no. I don't see why he should be tidying after people. I would rather him be at home than get a job.*

FORMAL CARER PERSPECTIVES

Formal carers at the ATCs had rather similar views, which can be summarized in terms of a number of key themes.

Formal carers felt that the higher-ability adults were not achieving their full potential and were capable of simple paid employment, independent living, sexual relationships and marriage.

> FORMAL CARER *I think there should be something else for the advanced ones at the ATC, some sort of work experience or independent living skills unit. Lots here have reached their full potential and have done for a long time.*

Although unemployment and lack of rights for disabled people were recognized as barriers; parental attitudes were seen as being the main problem. Three reasons were given for parental opposition to the adults becoming more autonomous. First, formal carers felt that parents were overprotective, i.e. not willing to accept 'normal' risks:

> FORMAL CARER *Parents, they think that they are very vulnerable and they can't sort of cope with situations like getting the right bus . . . There is a risk for everyone of crossing the road.*

Secondly, parents were seen as financially motivated to maintain adult dependence, e.g. because they would lose mobility allowances if adults learnt to use public transport:

> FORMAL CARER *Parents don't want to see them becoming independent as*

they will be losing their meal ticket with all their benefits. They would never outwardly state this but they do categorically say that they are not capable.

Thirdly, formal carers felt that communication with informal carers was often poor, that parents had understandable worries about safety, and were more willing to cooperate if training programmes were properly explained to them:

INTERVIEWER *Do you think there is enough communication between staff and parents?*

FORMAL CARER *No, I think there is a "them" and "us" feeling and they don't like being told what to do . . . If parents could find out what is going on they wouldn't be so scared.*

One formal carer felt that there was more than a communication problem, that normalization in the sense of paid employment or living independently were not necessarily what adults wanted:

FORMAL CARER *One lad, I got him a job doing some painting and after a few weeks I went to see him and he tells me that he hates painting. I asked him why he didn't tell us so he just says that he didn't like to. We do encourage people to do things that they probably don't want to do.*

Although informal carers were seen as the main obstacle to adults achieving their full potential, formal carers felt that there was nothing they could do if parents vetoed a particular form of training:

FORMAL CARER *Once parents say no here, though, we tend to leave it at that and not go back.*

Formal carers felt that parents of the more able adults were misusing the ATC and taking up places which were urgently needed for more disabled adults recently decanted into the community from institutional care:

FORMAL CARER *If they don't want them trained, they should take them out, the majority see it as a service to get the individual out of their home, a babysitting service.*

DISCUSSION

Comparison of the perspectives of adults, informal and formal carers shows that they view the role and purpose of the ATC very differently. Only a small minority of adults viewed the ATC as a place to learn, and most saw it as a place to work or were unsure why they were there. Their feelings towards the ATC varied, although all welcomed the opportunities it provided to meet friends and enjoy activities.

However, a number of the adults showed signs of frustration at limited opportunities in a variety of areas, including work, friendship, sexual relationships and independent living. In two cases there was overt rebellion. In other cases, frustration only emerged during lengthy interviewing. Adults had been pressured to accept certain ideas, e.g. that sexual relationships were 'rude' and that marriage was not a practical possibility.

Tension was evident between formal carers seeking to promote independence, and informal carers who wished to protect the adult from danger. This difference in perspective gave rise to the usual communication problems with each side tending to stereotype and accuse the other while failing to understand their point of view. Informal carers saw formal carers as trying to push adults beyond their capabilities without regard to their individual needs and limitations. Formal carers saw informal carers as overprotective, holding the adults back, sometimes for financial reasons. As a result, their views of the role of the ATC differed fundamentally from those of adults and informal carers. Formal carers saw the ATC essentially as a place which provided training for the adults to move on to less segregated, more demanding roles in the community. Informal carers and most adults saw the ATC as a permanent safe haven because it was outside a community which at best offered only a poor quality of life for adults and, at worst, was positively dangerous.

Policies designed to enhance autonomy for adults with learning difficulties must start from their aspirations. However, unless ways are found for adults, informal and formal carers to work together to promote adult autonomy, their aspirations will never be realized.

REFERENCES

Cathermole, M., Jahoda A. and Markova I. (1987) *Training for Independent Living in Mental Hospitals and ATCs*. Mimeograph, University of St. Andrews.

Flynn, M. and Saleem, J. (1986) Adults who are mentally handicapped and living with their parents: satisfaction and perceptions regarding their lives and circumstances. *Journal Of Mental Deficiency*, **30**, 379–87.

Heyman, B. and Huckle, S. (1993a) 'Normal' life in a hazardous world: how adults with learning difficulties and their carers cope with risks and dangers. *Disability, Handicap and Society*, **8**, 143–60.

Heyman, B. and Huckle, S. (1993b) Not worth the risk? Attitudes of adults with learning difficulties and their informal and formal carers to the hazards of everyday life. *Social Science and Medicine*, (in press)

Heyman, B. and Huckle, S. (1994) The needs of young adults with learning difficulties, in *Wicked Problems and Awkward Questions: User Perspectives on Community Health Care*, (ed B. Heyman), Chapman and Hall, London (in press).

Iano, R. (1970) Social class and parental evaluation of educable retarded children. *Education and Training of the Mentally Retarded*, **5**, 62–7.

Johnson, P. R. and Davies, R. (1989) Sexual attitudes of members of staff. *British Journal of Mental Subnormality*, **35**, 17–21.

Richardson, A. and Richie, J. (1989) *Developing Friendships: Enabling People with Learning Difficulties to Make and Maintain Friends*, Policy Studies Institute, London.

Sigelman, C., Budd, E., Spanhel, C. and Schoenrock, C. (1986) When in doubt say yes: acquiescence in interviews with mentally retarded persons. *Mental Retardation*, **19**, 53–8.

Strauss, A. and Corbin, J. (1990) *Basics of Qualitative Research*, Sage, London.

Winik, I., Zetlin, A. and Kaufman, S. Z. (1985) Adult mildly retarded persons and their parents: the relationship between involvement and adjustment. *Applied Research in Mental Retardation*, **6**, 409–19.

Wolfensberger, W. (1983) Social role valorization: a proposed new term for the principle of normalisation. *Mental Retardation*, **21**, 234–9.

PART THREE

The Way Forward

CHAPTER 11

Evaluating and developing practitioner research

Jan Reed and Colin Biott

INTRODUCTION

Throughout this book we have attempted to show how practitioner research can make a contribution to health care practice. We have discussed the special position of the practitioner researcher and the issues that arise from it, and drawn attention to the problems and pitfalls that this can bring. Many of these issues are not very different from those facing the non-practitioner researcher – many orthodox texts will address these issues – but we have made the case that practitioner knowledge, role and experience cast a particular light on the issue of human agency in research.

Throughout these discussions we have tried to avoid a naive stance which exalts the practitioner to some superior form of researcher – we do not believe that thoughtfulness, self-awareness and reflexivity will always accompany practitioner research, and so many of our comments have dwelt on problems and issues that must be tackled if practitioner research is to produce sound and meaningful studies. These comments, however, differ in many ways from traditional notions of validity, reliability, bias and generalization found in many textbooks, in that they reflect the awareness that practitioner research must be evaluated differently. This chapter attempts to put together and summarize these ideas about the evaluation of practitioner research, and then goes on to indicate how it may be developed further.

The argument for a different set of criteria for the evaluation of practitioner research arises from the combination of three ideas which are central to this book. First, we have argued for a constructionist view of research, which recognizes the part that the researcher plays in constructing knowledge. Secondly, we have argued that the researcher in practitioner research has particular knowledge and understanding which profoundly affects the way in which research is conducted.

Thirdly, we have argued that practitioner research has a particular type of motivation and aims, distinct from the rationale and goals of other types of research.

If these three points are accepted then it follows that the criteria used in non-practitioner research, which assume either naivety or neutrality or both on the part of the researcher, are not appropriate in practitioner research. If these criteria are used, then the value of practitioner research will be lost amid accusations of impressionistic anecdotalism, and strenuous attempts to refute these criticisms will serve only to obscure the particular nature of practitioner research still further.

It is probably worthwhile here to consider traditional research evaluation in more detail, and to debate the problems in using these criteria in practitioner research. One important question is that of validity, which is essentially a question about whether the research measures or studies what it claims to. Validity can be and has been divided into many types, for example construct and concept validity, but essentially it is about the 'soundness' of the research and the extent to which it can be held to represent reality, and whether there is anything about the research that may distort reality. These ideas, of course, rest upon the assumption that there is a 'reality' which can be represented; in other words, there is a reality which exists independent of our experience of it and so can be 'captured' by the right research approach.

This notion of validity is therefore problematic in itself, but when applied to practitioner research it becomes even more difficult to address. This is largely because the representation of reality that is produced by research is partly evaluated by the degree to which the findings are independent of the researcher, and thus accessible to all. The question is asked, implicitly or explicitly: 'If someone else had done this research, would they have got the same results?' If we accept that the position of the practitioner researcher is not replicable within a study, i.e. that someone else could not have done the research, or if they had they would have had to conduct it differently, then it is impossible to answer 'yes' to this question. Because of this, the researcher immediately becomes an agent of distortion.

Perhaps a more appropriate view of the process of validation is proposed by Maturana (1991), when he argues that one of the operations that must be performed on explanations is 'The presentation of the experience (phenomena) to be explained in terms of what a standard observer must do in his or her domain of experience (praxis of living) to experience it' (p. 32). Maturana goes on to outline further operations in the process of validation, which can be summarized as the reformulation of the phenomena as a generative mechanism and the deduction from this of other experiences which the standard observer should have as a result of this generative mechanism. Maturana's view is that the researcher cannot do more than this: describe their experience under the conditions in which they experienced it, suggest ways in which others might experience it and identify different or other experiences that the 'standard observer' (another researcher) might have.

Clearly this is not a view based on traditional notions of replication, but it does place on the researcher some responsibility for generating further research by others. This form of validity, which later in this chapter we have called 'catalytic validity', does not assume that research can be simply replicated and that its value or validity lies in the extent to which this can be done, but that it can and should contribute to further research by others. The researcher therefore has a responsibility to others who follow, to give them as clear an account of the research as possible, including their practitioner identity, to help them in their research.

Another related criterion of research which is often debated is reliability, in other words the question about whether the results of a study have been derived through approaches which are consistent, or whether they are subject to vagaries of data collection. Reliability is closely linked to validity but is perhaps more narrow in definition, usually referring to data collection tools rather than the entire study. In practitioner research, debates about reliability can have relevance to the methods used in the research, for example questionnaires or observation schedules, but where the main research tools are the researchers themselves then this becomes more problematic.

One of the checks which is often suggested in research, particularly where observation tools are used, is a check on interrater reliability. In traditional research it is quite a normal procedure to get more than one researcher to complete an observation or interview schedule, and compare results. The degree to which data recording is consistent is the measure of the reliability of the tool. In practitioner research this may well be possible in some cases, but in others it will be impossible or meaningless. The presence of another researcher in clinical settings can be in itself a threat to reliability and, in cases where the research tool is the researcher, we would not expect the researcher to be able to ensure consistency simply by comparing interpretations with someone else, who brings with them their own vagaries. Val Pirie's chapter in this book (Chapter 5) illustrates these problems.

Reliability checks in practitioner research, therefore, might be more usefully thought of as exercises in 'sounding out' interpretations. Using a colleague, friend or supervisor to examine data, rather than data collection, is undeniably useful, provided that the relationship is one which produces fruitful debate. As individuals we are all subject to changes in mood or attentiveness and someone else can often identify such inconsistencies better than we can ourselves. This takes us away somewhat from the notion of research (and particularly qualitative research) as being an purely individual endeavour which is a completely private process, and instead opens it up to more public debate. This is an alarming prospect for some, who are reluctant to expose their tender studies to the frosts of public debate, but the result may be a more robust plant.

Debates on validity and reliability are both ultimately concerned with the notion of bias and how this can be controlled. Bias, in its statistical sense, is an issue concerning the representativeness of samples and data – a sample can be biased towards a particular group if sampling strategies are flawed (for example if the sample has not included a full range of the population) and data can be biased if tools are not well designed (for example a questionnaire that asks leading questions, or encourages some responses and prevents others).

Bias is problematic in research partly because it limits the extent to which results can be generalized, and generalized knowledge is important not only in the way that it can be applied to a population wider than the research sample, but also in the way that results can contribute to theory development and testing. This notion of the desirability of generalization is again at odds with practitioner research. The logic behind generalization rests partly on the assumption that good research will use random samples (whose representativeness will be amenable to calculation) which are of a sufficient size to justify the mathematical exercise of extending sample results to the larger population.

Most practitioner research uses small samples, largely because the practitioner researcher has limited time and resources to extend the study beyond their immediate practice. This immediately reduces the worth of practitioner research in traditional academic terms. If it were possible to widen samples then these criticisms might be met, but something would also be lost in terms of practitioner research. Data collected in an area of practice that one knows well are of a very different quality from those collected in a wider field, not only because they lose the fine detail possible in small studies, but because the immediate concerns and intimate understanding of the practitioner researcher are lost.

We would therefore suggest that, rather than thinking about sample bias and generalization, it is more appropriate and productive to think about theoretical sampling and usefulness. Both of these ideas have been discussed elsewhere in this book (see Chapter 3), but they are worth addressing here too. Theoretical sampling (an idea first explicitly discussed by Glaser and Strauss, 1967) is a form of sampling in which phenomena or people are chosen for the study not under the strictures of randomness, but because they are the most fruitful avenues for the development of theory. In practitioner research, where the theoretical understanding desired is a small-scale analysis of specific phenomena, rather than grand theory statements couched in universal terms, it makes sense to sample the phenomena in the environment in which they first came to the attention of the researcher. In other words, sampling in practitioner research might not be about representativeness but about uniqueness.

Talking about usefulness rather than generalization again casts a different light on the evaluation of practitioner research. If practitioner research is presented in such a way that the reader can understand the particular features of the research setting, then it becomes more possible to compare and contrast those features with the reader's own practice setting and for the reader to identify similarities and differences which would determine the extent or way in which research could be used there.

Bias also has a commonsense formulation, however, derived from the way that people talk about bias in everyday talk. Bias here becomes another variant of subjectivity, and it is in this way that it becomes a threat to the reliability and validity of research. The argument here is that subjectivity, or bias, leads researchers into partisan interpretations which are value-laden.

The fear of being seen to have values and therefore denounced as a biased researcher has led many researchers, not only practitioner researchers, to deny that they have them. For all researchers, however, this denial is necessarily false, which we can see if we look at just one stage of the research process, deciding to undertake a study. For non-practitioner researchers who belong to a scientific or academic community their choice of study will be influenced by what is valued in this community as being good research. Good research may be seen as 'objective', and therefore their formulation of the research question will be couched in such terms, perhaps as a dispassionate review of the literature; their methods will be chosen for their scientific respectability and their results will be derived from scientific procedures for analysis. Even if the researcher has no personal interest in the research – say they have taken a research job on a project simply in order to earn a living – then an implicit part of their job, and the way that their success will be measured, is in the way they adhere to the principle of scientific research and objectivity. In this way objectivity itself becomes a value, or, as Barthes (1986) has argued, objectivity is simply a special case of interpretation.

Values (or subjective views) are perhaps more readily apparent in practitioner research. Improving patient care is an important driving force behind practitioner research, determining the choice of topic, the way the area is studied and the way any findings are presented. To remove values from practitioner research seems like a contradiction in terms – without such motivation practitioner research is no different from other forms of study.

Values and motivation in practitioner research can be extended beyond the immediate benefit of the patient. As in education, we are starting to see the debate about top-down and bottom-up developments increasingly portrayed as an issue about the best way of facilitating a caring and conscientious approach to practice. The argument for practitioner research that we make here is, in part, based on the notion that it will develop a reflective approach to practice which will go beyond the immediate research project. This is not, therefore, a disinterested academic debate about the reliability or validity of different research methods, but rather about the way in which things that we value can be achieved.

The things we value in research are inextricably connected to the things we value in practice, for example imaginative approaches, collaborative practices and the sensitive understanding of contexts. If we accept the worth of values as a catalyst for practice and research, then we may be able to begin to identify the hallmarks of strong practitioner research as research which embodies these values, rather than the values of objectivity which have prevailed in traditional science. These traditional values are often the sources of unease and criticism of practitioner research, even among those who undertake it, and can lead to elaborate arguments for and justifications of practitioner research which use inappropriate ideas of rigour. The result is a lack of attention to the special aims of practitioner research, and a position which portrays it as a second-best alternative to 'proper' science. It is being suggested here, therefore, that practitioner values should form part of the way in which practitioner research is evaluated.

If we abandon, or at least query, traditional criteria for good research, however, we are left in an unproductive position where we come close to saying that 'anything goes'. This does not advance the position of practitioner research in our own eyes or in the eyes of others, but more importantly it does not allow us to develop any further. This problem is evident in many of the chapters in this book, where researchers felt unable to identify appropriate ways of evaluating what they had done, or make decisions about what they should do, given that they had recognized that traditional research prescriptions did not fit their study. What is apparent in these chapters, however, is that the researchers were all motivated by the practitioner values they held and the commitment they had to developing patient care. These values seem a useful starting point for an attempt to identify more precisely some criteria which could be used to evaluate and guide practitioner research.

'STRONG' AND 'WEAK' PRACTITIONER RESEARCH

Taking this idea further, we shall outline and discuss a set of guiding principles which might be used to distinguish strong practitioner research from weaker forms. We do not use the terms 'good' and 'bad' research, as these imply absolute states, whereas we think it more likely that research studies will neither be all 'good' nor all 'bad'. We recognize, however, that using the terms strong and weak creates similar problems, although these terms do convey a more appropriate sense of relativity. It must also be appreciated that these terms are used in relation to practitioner research rather than any other form – we are not claiming that the criteria we propose fit all types of research, nor that all research should address these criteria.

The list below sets out what might be proposed as idealized criteria for practitioner research. These are derived from the inherent values of practitioner research and the particular position and knowledge of practitioner researchers and, as such, present a very different view of the criteria traditionally used to evaluate research. Practitioner research could be evaluated according to the extent to which it is:

- integral with the practice of health care;
- a social process undertaken with colleagues;
- educative for all participants in the projects;
- imbued with an integral development dimension:
- focused upon aspects of practice in which the researcher has some control and can initiate change;
- able to identify and explore sociopolitical and historical factors affecting practice;
- able to open up value issues for critical enquiry and discussion;
- designed so as to give a say to all participants;
- able to exercise the professional imagination and enhance the capacity of participants to interpret everyday action in the work setting;
- able to integrate personal and professional learning;
- likely to yield insights which can be conveyed in a form which make them worthy of interest to a wider audience.

1. Strong practitioner research, we believe, is integral with the practice of health care itself. We base this view upon our assumption that health care has a research dimension in which the practitioner carries out tasks such as asking questions, listening, observing and interpreting as an everyday aspect of the job. Part of the work, for instance, involves trying to see things from the perspective of the patients or clients. For this reason it is necessary to enquire in order to do health care work. In its strong form, practitioner research does not require that the person stops practising in order to carry out a project, or that it should be very different from the type of 'attentive practice' which marks good patient care.

This attentive practice (some may prefer the term 'reflective practice') involves paying careful attention to events in practice, and reflecting on them. Attentive practice can be the motivation for research, as the practitioner identifies an issue that requires further study, or it can form part of the research data as the skills of observation used in practice are used in research. Strong practitioner research should be an extension of good practice and not an activity alien to the practice role.

2.   Practitioner research is a social process undertaken with colleagues to explore and try to build shared meanings and understandings together. Negotiation is a central part of health care, and multiprofessional teams in particular can benefit from collaborative enquiry into their working practices over such things as what counts as care.

3.   Practitioner research is essentially educative, in that it offers opportunities for all participants to learn collectively through the research processes themselves. Because the participants are colleagues, patients or families, it follows that they will not be relegated to the status of mere research subjects, but become research participants. The strength of projects will be related partly to the extent of genuine rather than token involvement. The weakest version of learning from research is to be merely told of findings. The strongest versions involve all participants in taking decisions about what evidence to collect, how to collect it, how to interpret it and what actions to take in the light of those interpretations. Furthermore, people in the studies will share, in different ways and depending upon practical feasibility and appropriateness, the tasks of data collection and interpretation.

This moves away from the 'solitary genius' image of research in which ideas are the property of individuals with special abilities, and moves research into the domain of public debate. This is not to suggest that research becomes a matter for committees, with the role of the individual suppressed, but it changes the research from a monologue to a dialogue in which ideas are not simply presented to an audience, but are generated and developed collaboratively.

4.   Practitioner research has an integral development dimension, linked to the idea of collaboration. Through their engagement with analysis and discovery, people in the studies will be motivated and supported to try out new practices, which will grow out of ideas raised. The new practices should be seen as provisional and requiring further critical scrutiny rather than being conclusive. Even though decisions are made the talking and enquiring continues, a form of validity very close to that proposed by Lather (1986) when she discussed catalytic validity. Catalytic validity concerns the power of the research to stimulate debate rather than conclude it.

5.   Practitioner research should lead to action rather than to pious claims about prediction and generalization, or to the attaching of blame

to others. This has implications for the design of studies, as they will have a clear focus upon aspects of practice over which the person initiating the research has some control. This means that it would be appropriate for a health care practitioner to make a study of practice in a number of hospitals for which they have direct responsibility, but it would be a 'cop out' (in practitioner research terms) for someone who worked solely within one unit to claim that their study showed that something needed doing on a scale beyond the scope of their own practice. This is not simply a debate about 'going beyond the data' but is about being satisfied with realizable goals. If the concern is about improving practice, then this will be necessarily constrained by the context in which it occurs, and the research should reflect this and include a description of these constraints sufficient to allow the reader to understand it. As we have discussed above, the goal is to produce useful rather than generalizable data.

The notions of good research as being widely generalizable, so often found in traditional science, exercise a strong influence on the way in which studies are written up, and practitioners can sometimes feel embarrassed about the localized nature of their study. The temptation is to attempt greater academic credibility by claiming widespread or even universal relevance of results. This is not only spurious but is not particularly useful; indeed, it is almost insulting to the reader. Giving a detailed description of a localized research setting, as we have argued above, allows readers to make an informed choice about the relevance of the research to their own practice. It then becomes possible for the reader to identify commonalties and differences between the research setting and their own field, and use the research findings accordingly.

What is perhaps more important than the size of the study (and sometimes even more important than results) is the level and quality of the theoretical analysis that it contains. A rigorous and critical analysis of concepts in the study data which leads to theoretical development is perfectly possible, and indeed often more manageable in a small study than in a large one. This type of theoretical development has tradition- ally belonged to the inductive rather than the deductive approach to theory, i.e. small-scale studies have been viewed as ways of generating theory inductively, which can then be tested deductively using large- scale studies. The subsequent deductive testing of theory is traditionally devoted to hypothesis testing and attempts to refute theories, but in practitioner research it may be more useful to think of theory testing as an effort to find out where, when and under what circumstances theor- ies are useful to practice. The goal may not be the wholesale rejection of theories but modification and qualification – goals which suggest that small-scale studies may be equally useful for theory modification as well as theory generation. Most texts on research methods depict qualitative methodology and small-scale studies as a source of theory generation rather than testing. Chapter 4, however, makes the case for using qualitative methods to test theory and values underpinning research findings within a clinical context.

6.   Practitioner research should increase understanding of the sociopolitical factors affecting professional practice. Although its prime purpose is to investigate and develop the practices of the setting in which the person works, it should avoid being blinkered and parochial. Some aspects of practice are deeply embedded in the history of our professions and it may be necessary to identify and come to terms with taken-for-granted and habituated customs in order to reorientate ourselves to pose more penetrating questions. In this way practitioner research can embrace the sociopolitical issues which are, after all, an integral part of the practice context. Two chapters in this book have described research which was aware of and affected by sociopolitical issues: Chapter 7, where Ruth McKeown found that the project that she was managing and researching was fundamentally changed by policy decisions, and Chapter 8, where Jean Davies' experiences as a midwife led her to study housing patterns in the area in which she worked, and to see them as significant to her practice.

7.   Practitioner research in its strongest form should involve close scrutiny of key concepts and values which underpin and shape practices. Eraut (1985), for example, has drawn attention to how school teachers have 'rhetorics of justification' to talk about teaching. For this reason, groups of teachers will often rehearse familiar points and gain easy agreements from colleagues when discussing their experiences. In order to explore value issues in a fruitful way, it is useful to have actual evidence available for shared analysis by the group. The next step is to identify the concepts which are of concern rather than make judgements about personal stances. In a health care setting this may mean that a group should focus upon the concept of, say, individualized care (a nebulous notion indeed). To concentrate on what this entails will open possibilities for another stage of evidence collection which will widen and at the same time sharpen the orientation of an enquiry. Practitioner research, therefore, should not unquestioningly perpetuate clichés about practice, but should make them part of the enquiry.

8.   Practitioner research extends the criteria for judging everyday practice during the course of that practice and enhances the capacities of interpretation. The processes of practitioner research utilize professional imagination and educate the professional sensibilities. For this reason,

projects which begin from a sense of unease and which ask the question 'What is happening here?' are often preferable to those that ask questions about effectiveness. The latter are more likely to become instrumental projects, rather like the kinds of limited evaluation studies that attach priority to majority opinions and suggest solutions for implementation. Practitioner research takes on board the idea that there may be no easy or definitive answers to the problems of practice, and resists the temptation to produce these answers at the expense of asking difficult questions. This requires acknowledgement of the idea that the world of practice is constantly changing and constantly uncertain.

In developing these criteria we have tried to reflect some of the ideas that underpin the notion of the practitioner researcher, i.e. practitioners who are researching their practice. These are not simply ideas about how the practitioner researcher is disadvantaged in relation to the traditional academic researcher in terms of their lack of distance or objectivity, but of how these characteristics might equally well be construed as advantages for this particular kind of research. The differences lie in the person of the researcher, in their knowledge and goals, and we have argued that it is only relatively recently that such personal characteristics have been acknowledged in traditional research. If we begin to think about research as a personalized activity, then these characteristics have profound implications for the conduct of research studies.

These criteria are based on the discussions of the knowledge base and goals of the practitioner researcher contained in the first four chapters of this book. What we have done here is to attempt to develop a set of criteria for conducting and evaluating practitioner research which reflects the particular nature of this type of enquiry. These criteria, however, will not fit all research done by people who are practitioners, because some will prefer or wish to take a more traditional path, and there is a great deal to be said for multiple perspectives and approaches on issues as important as health care – we are not discounting the usefulness of health care practitioners leaving their current work, say through secondment, to work on research projects. We also accept that some people will seek to study topics of interest across regions or in unfamiliar settings, say through part-time courses which give them opportunities to learn a range of research methods or to extend their knowledge in ways that would be difficult within the limitations of their own work environments. Some may even wish to train as professional researchers with a view to leaving direct employment in health care.

For those who use traditional approaches, the criteria we set forth here are not necessarily appropriate: traditional criteria are more relevant. By the same token, however, traditional research evaluation is not the best way to examine practitioner research. These debates about evaluation and criteria are extremely important to the development of practitioner research, and not simply as a defence against critics. By looking at the hallmarks of strong practitioner research we can come closer to understanding, expressing and articulating what it is about, and what it can offer health care.

FUTURE DEVELOPMENTS

The future development of practitioner research as a distinct form of research depends much upon the recognition of its potential contribution to health care among practitioners, other types of researcher and those who can give support to research studies: managers and funding bodies. These three groups are all important: practitioners because they are the people who will do the research and use it most directly; other researchers because they will accept practitioner research not as inferior but as a different way of doing things; and those who support this research because they can give it the resources it needs.

The support of these three groups is, of course, interrelated. Practitioners, managers and funding bodies derive at least some of their criteria from those used in non-practitioner research (this is particularly true of funding bodies), which means that the recognition of other researchers of practitioner research as a valid form of enquiry is important. To promote this recognition, however, we must be prepared to engage in debate with the traditional research community and be prepared to defend our position. To this end we need to be clear about our own position, and hopefully this book is a move towards such clarification.

At another level, however, practitioner research is evaluated by practitioners and managers in terms of its usefulness in informing practice, and this is congruent with many of the ideas that we have set out here. For practitioners, however, the usefulness will be in part dependent on their own confidence in using research creatively rather than mechanistically – practitioner research, as we have argued, is more about generating debate than solving it, and will not provide easy prescriptions for others to follow. This suggests that Hunt's (1981) category of research which 'tells people what they should do' will be less prominent than research which 'tells people what they can try'.

This development, however, requires some changes in the way that research is tackled in the training and education of health care practitioners, particularly how research is approached. Developing a curriculum that incorporates qualitative and quantitative approaches, and which also addresses the philosophical foundations of feminist, action and new-paradigm research goes some way towards facilitating a creative use of research in practice, and those courses which are designed to facilitate research skills in practitioners can also incorporate these ideas. More generally, however, the principles of reflective practice, used throughout the curriculum can be used to foster a critical and thoughtful approach to theory and research (Reed and Procter, 1993).

For managers, practitioner research may sit uncomfortably with ideas of rational management which have until recently been prevalent in management theory. Rational management, which was based on a 'scientistic' notion of the world derived from objective science, has little in common with ideas about artistry, intuition and small-scale theory. Rational managers like their theories big and their knowledge quantified.

New developments in management theory, and particularly in evaluation research, indicate that rational management is being challenged by a less scientistic approach. This may mean that practitioner research becomes a valued part of organizational learning, which is based on the view of organizations as organic and naturally evolving rather than mechanical and subject to periodic overhauls. Practitioner research fits more comfortably with the idea of evolutionary change, and therefore may gain more resources and support in the future.

Talking about practitioner research and resources seems to be an anomaly, as throughout this book we have portrayed practitioner research as being relatively cheap. Practitioner researchers typically conduct small studies and data collection is often a relatively minor extension of the practice role. It is tempting, therefore, to sell the idea of practitioner research as being very cheap.

Practitioner research, however, cannot be seen simply as a series of separate studies, isolated from the world in which they take place, and although we have argued that practitioner research can have an impact on the ethos of health care, we can also argue that the ethos of health care has an impact on practitioner research.

If the changes in management styles and approaches that we have tentatively identified are to support practitioner research, then this support will have to be more than simply financial. Funding a practitioner research study is all very well, but if organizations do not have mechanisms for using these studies as part of a debate about developments in health care, they will remain the private hobbies of those who conduct them. This problem has long been known in educational research, where teachers have for some time been encouraged and funded to conduct research as part of the 'teacher as researcher' movement, but have had problems in integrating their research into decisions about educational policy.

Adelman (1993), in his discussion of practitioner research in education, says that it remains to be seen whether participatory research can influence social and educational policy in technocratic bureaucracies. He suggests that the recent emphasis upon individual reflectivity will not promote democratic participation, and he advocates the 'essential inclusion of group and institutional relationships' (Adelman, 1993, p.21) if we are to improve practice in the context of current constraints. Elliott (1993) also wishes to see a continuation of 'the collaborative reconstruction of the professional culture of teachers through the development of discursive consciousness' (Elliott, 1993, p.185). He argues that it is difficult to make changes in the practices of schools without taking into account the need to bring about corresponding changes in all the interlocking subsystems. For this reason, he wishes to see a widening of school-based action research so that school administrators, parents, employers and teachers are engaged in discourse grounded in data from practice.

The parallels between the debates in health care research and educational research are fairly clear. There has been a concern in both fields about the gaps between theory and practice, and about the way in which theory is being developed and transmitted. In health care research, however, the solutions have until recently been sought in terms of individual researchers and projects, and the search has used orthodox criteria about the best way to conduct research. Practitioner research, which takes a collaborative approach, does not conform to these criteria. It is possible, therefore, that under current funding criteria practitioner research could be construed as 'development of practice' or 'service evaluation' rather than research, and therefore lose out on access to funding. This could create particular dilemmas for practitioners in that recent strategy documents have emphasized the importance of applied research to the health service, but continued to define this research according to the orthodox criteria. Those proposals which, to the practitioner, seem most likely to improve practice, may be given low ratings by funding bodies because they do not look as if they will produce generalizable results, one of the hallmarks of traditional research.

This suggests that the debate should be widened to challenge traditional definitions of a 'research culture' and the way that it can be developed. The experience of educational practitioner research indicates that there is a need to develop mechanisms for discourse within health care organizations if practitioner research in health care is to develop further and have a positive impact on practice. In health care research, however, this is likely to be particularly difficult given the multidisciplinary nature of health care settings and the overriding power of the medical profession. In health care settings practitioner research will need to take on board political and organizational contexts as an integral part of study, and also as an integral part of the dissemination and presentation of research. With current disparities in the distribution of power, resources and status this could be extremely difficult to achieve.

Although health care practitioners may have been taught about change strategies these often assume a degree of power and control beyond the scope of the individual practitioner, and fail to recognize the complexity of health care systems from a practitioner rather than a managerial perspective. There is a danger that the complexities of multidisciplinary negotiations required to bring about changes in the distribution of power will prevent the development of collaborative research across professional boundaries. Consequently, practitioners may well have to narrow their focus to their own practice, thus perpetuating current divisions and divides in the health service and maintaining the current medical orientation of the service.

Practitioner research is therefore caught at the centre of an ideological debate about the nature of research. Adopting the principles of traditional research will provide rich rewards in terms of funding and status, but is unlikely to have any impact on issues central to their own practice development. This highlights the need for those responsible for the funding of research to take a critical look at the criteria being used, and to decide whether those criteria are going to produce the type of policy directives required if health services are to move from a medically orientated perspective to one which deals more appropriately with changing health care needs.

This is essentially the motivation for this book – to begin to clarify the particular position of the practitioner researcher and the nature of the research that they do. It is, however, only a beginning and much of what has been written here is exploratory rather than definitive. This is the way it should be, because premature conclusions will inhibit development much more than tentative propositions. Our hope is that this book will engender much debate and further exploration of the issues that have been raised.

There are some areas which clearly require further exploration. In particular, we need to know more about practitioner knowledge – we can only argue here that it must provide a foundation for practitioner research and we can indicate ways in which this might happen and cite specific examples from our experience. A fuller understanding of professional knowledge, however, will help us to take this further. We also need to engage in methodological debates and studies in which the practitioner role is explicitly recognized. At present most methodological texts and papers concentrate on the issues in the methods themselves, rather than on the way the researcher identity can affect them.

Ironically, perhaps, these developments may not arise from practitioner research alone – similar endeavours are taking place in many areas of research, including traditional scientific fields. This observation is not made grudgingly – we recognize the value of different research approaches according to their different aims. What we are arguing here is that practitioner research is different from other forms of research, simply because practitioner researchers have different goals and experiences from non-practitioner researchers. The question of whether practitioner research is a good thing or a bad thing, or whether it is better than other forms of research is in many ways secondary to this observation.

Our position is that practitioner research happens and will continue to happen more and more as practitioners engage in research, and we would argue that the time has come to acknowledge this and to develop methodologies which are congruent with its aims.

REFERENCES

Adelman, C. (1993) Kurt Lewin and the origins of action research. *Educational Action Research*, **1**(1), 2–24.

Barthes, R. (1986) *The Rustle of Language*, Hill and Wang, New York.

Elliott, J. (1993) What have we learned from action research in school-based evaluation? *Educational Action Research*, **1**(1), 175.

Eraut, M. (1985) Knowledge creation and use in professional contexts. *Studies in Higher Education*, **10**(2), 117–33.

Glaser, B. G. and Strauss, A. L. (1967) *The Discovery of Grounded Theory: Strategies for Qualitative Research*, Aldine, Chicago.

Hunt, J. (1981) Indications for nursing practice: the use of research findings. *Journal of Advanced Nursing*, **6**, 189–94.

Lather, P. (1986) Research as praxis. *Harvard Educational Review*, **56**(3), 257–77.

Maturana, H. R. (1991) Science and daily life: the ontology of scientific explanations, in *Research and Reflexivity*, (ed F. Steier), Sage, London, pp. 30–52.

Reed, J. and Procter, S. (1993) *Nurse Education: A Reflective Approach*, Edward Arnold, London.

Index

Page numbers appearing in **bold** refer to figures and page numbers appearing in *italic* refer to tables.